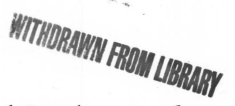

Bioethics beyond the Headlines

Bioethics beyond the Headlines

Who Lives? Who Dies? Who Decides?

Albert R. Jonsen

ROWMAN & LITTLEFIELD PUBLISHERS, INC.
Lanham · Boulder · New York · Toronto · Oxford

ROWMAN & LITTLEFIELD PUBLISHERS, INC.

Published in the United States of America
by Rowman & Littlefield Publishers, Inc.
A wholly owned subsidiary of The Rowman & Littlefield Publishing Group, Inc.
4501 Forbes Boulevard, Suite 200, Lanham, Maryland 20706
www.rowmanlittlefield.com

PO Box 317
Oxford
OX2 9RU, UK

Copyright © 2005 by Rowman & Littlefield Publishers, Inc.

British Library Cataloguing in Publication Information Available

Library of Congress Cataloging-in-Publication Data

Jonsen, Albert R.
  Bioethics beyond the headlines : who lives? who dies? who decides? / Albert R. Jonsen.
    p. cm.
  Includes bibliographical references and index.
  ISBN 0-7425-4523-7 (cloth : alk. paper) — ISBN 0-7425-4524-5 (pbk. : alk. paper)
  1. Medical ethics. 2. Bioethics.
  [DNLM: 1. Bioethical Issues. WB 60 J81b 2005] I. Title.
  R724.J655 2005
  174.2—dc22   2005006742

Printed in the United States of America

∞™ The paper used in this publication meets the minimum requirements of American
National Standard for Information Sciences—Permanence of Paper for Printed Library
Materials, ANSI/NISO Z39.48-1992.

Contents

Introduction

"In New Tests for Fetal Defects, Agonizing Choices for Parents"

*T*his 2004 headline story details the number of diagnostic tests that can now be performed on a fetus during pregnancy. Expectant parents can learn that their baby will be born with cystic fibrosis, a cleft palate, a brain cyst, Kleinfelder's sydrome, and some four hundred fifty other conditions. Some of these conditions, such as Tay-Sachs disease, bring the baby to a devastating and early death; others, such as Down's syndrome, mean a lifetime with mental disability. The article describes the agony of parents who receive this unwelcome news. They must, it states, face the decision of whether to abort. It then states, "The wider range and earlier timing of prenatal tests are raising concerns among some bioethicists" and quotes a "bioethicist," who says "By putting [these tests] out there as something everyone must do, the profession communicates that these are conditions that everyone must avoid."[1]

"Bioethicists" first appeared in the 1970s. For about two decades, they hid shyly in the pages of a few specialized books and articles about the arcane realms of medicine, science, and philosophy. Recently, they have broken into the public media, appearing in stories about whether a doctor should hasten a patient's death, whether a scientist should create a human embryo in order to do research on it, or whether new knowledge about the genetic makeup of the human race should be used to shape stronger, healthier, smarter persons. In the story cited above, a bioethicist expresses concern about a "slippery slide from prenatal science to eugenics." In these news stories, bioethicists are

1

quoted alongside scientists or activists or ministers. Who are these bioethicists? Do their comments carry any authority, as does the scientific knowledge
of a prominent biochemist discussing biochemistry or the statement of a
church leader discussing doctrine?

This book is an introduction to the work that bioethicists do. It attempts
to explain to the curious reader some of the problems grouped under the title
of bioethics and some responses to those problems that bioethicists propose.
It hopes to show that the brief (often inaccurate) comments that journalists
snatch from bioethicists for their articles or interviews can be placed against
a wide background of ideas and arguments. And, because bioethics has had
influence beyond the academic world in which it was born, this book follows
some of the field's ideas into public policy, medical practice, and law.

There are many books on bioethics written for scholars in the field, for
students taking bioethics courses in college or professional school, and for
health care practitioners seeking guidance in their work. Many bioethics articles appear in specialized journals. Those books and articles explain bioethics
or some particular bioethical issue in the exact, detailed fashion preferred in
academic or professional writing. This book is written to make bioethics accessible to any curious reader. If such a reader is intrigued enough to delve
more deeply, I note at the end of each chapter some books, journals, or web-
sites that can open the way. I regularly cite entries in the *Encyclopedia of
Bioethics*.[2] This multivolume work, found in most libraries, contains concise
entries on all of the topics mentioned in this book. I also cite a major textbook, *The Principles of Biomedical Ethics*, by Tom Beauchamp and James Childress,[3] which provides carefully detailed arguments on the issues. I occasionally cite my own book, *The Birth of Bioethics*, when it is useful to know the
history of the issues.[4] Each of these books contains a multitude of references
to further studies. I rarely cite articles, of which there are thousands, because
it would be difficult to limit the list, pick the best, or cite the most current.

The title of this book, *Bioethics beyond the Headlines: Who Lives? Who
Dies? Who Decides?* is easy to explain. The "bio" in bioethics means "life," coming from the Greek word *bios*. The subject of bioethics is life but not as described in the biosciences, which attempt to discern the chemical, physical,
and environmental processes that sustain living beings. Bioethics is about life
as a value, worthy to be fostered by human decisions and actions. The phrase
"value of life" is a large generalization. We recognize that life can be pitted
against life, that life is created, grows, and deteriorates, and that our choices
about reproduction, medicine, and science can affect the ways in which the
value we place on life is manifested. We must ask many deep questions about
our choices. Bioethics is a scholarly attempt to collect those questions and to
seek answers.

We encounter life not in general but in particular living beings: the baby born prematurely whose lungs are hardly ready to breath air; the old man, long demented, who contracts pneumonia; the two candidates for a single transplantable heart; a patient racked with cancer pain asking to end life; the many sick persons awaiting new treatments that may save thousands but endanger some or be too costly for others. These and like situations force us to ask the questions that subtitle this book: Who lives? Who dies? Who decides? Patients, their families and friends, doctors, nurses, and social workers face these agonizing questions. Judges, lawyers, and legislators are sometimes forced to consider them. The public, whose attention is caught by a dramatic instance of life in question, wonders whether there are any answers. This book is written for all these people.

Bioethics beyond the Headlines is a primer in bioethics, an introduction to the topics and discussions that engage bioethicists. But a primer is not merely a first book; it should also "prime" the interest of the reader, prepare the mind for a more expansive venture into these issues by starting with a small dose. I do not provide the detailed arguments that might be found in the textbooks or scholarly treatises. Many bioethical questions involve convoluted philosophical arguments. I apologize to my readers for simplifying these. I do not try to cover all of the questions raised by bioethicists. I simply offer this as a starter, pointing toward how these questions have arisen and how some scholars have attempted to answer them. Although this is not a history of bioethics, this book will relate some historic debates and describe some of the signal cases that have stimulated them. Without reference to past ideas and events, it is difficult to understand contemporary opinion. My exposition of many topics begins with a minidebate between two pioneers of bioethics, Joseph Fletcher (1905–1991) and Paul Ramsey (1913–1988). These minidebates between two scholars who frequently stood at opposite ends of issues nicely set the stage for further debate by their successors. Sometimes, subsequent argument has not gotten much beyond their positions; at other times, bioethicists have raised new points and made different arguments. And the formulation of the ethical problem has shifted with experience and scientific innovation.

Readers will find more questions than answers in these pages. That is very much the nature of ethical debate. Often the questions circle around the problem without settling into resolution. Still, bioethical debate has reached some stopping points. Bioethicists, while rarely unanimous in their opinion on anything, are close to general agreement on some matters: most reject involuntary euthanasia, harvesting organs without consent, selling organs, cloning humans, treating permanently unconscious persons as dead, and treating or experimenting on persons without consent. Their opinions on these issues have not infrequently found their way into public opinion, health policy, medical practice, and law. Finally, bioethics is a moving subject, racing along as fast as (or perhaps just a bit behind) rapid scientific and medical advances. The media constantly portray "medical miracles" and novel cases, and bioethical commentary often follows. A book like this aspires to be up to date, but surely, it will not be as current as the media (it will be more accurate, I hope). I have tried to lay out the principal issues as they stand in 2005. A book like this appearing in 2015 will certainly look quite different.

This book is divided into four parts. Part I is an essay on the meaning and origins of bioethics and its relation to the broader academic field of ethics. Parts II through IV are divided into topics rather than chapters. Each topic represents a major issue that appears in standard bioethics. Part II, "Clinical Bioethics," deals with questions of bioethics that arise in the practice of clinical medicine. These are issues that physicians and their patients encounter as they work together to diagnose and treat disease. Part III, "Scientific Bioethics," discusses the ethical questions associated with medical progress. The first topic in this part, "Research with Humans: Experimentation, Autonomy, and Benefits to Others," deals with the search for progress by engaging humans as research subjects. The next three topics concern sciences that are still moving from the laboratory to the clinic, namely, genetics, neuroscience, and "regenerative medicine." These sciences pose unique ethical problems. Although some of these have already appeared in clinical practice, many of the ethical problems posed in these fields are anticipated rather than actual; they are foreseen as the possible consequences of further scientific discovery.

Finally, part IV, "The Wider World of Bioethics," treats topics that are larger than either the clinic or the laboratory, namely, the problems of access to health care, the place of animals in medical research, and the cultural setting in which bioethical problems arise. A final topic, "Environmental Ethics," presents a field of ethics not usually included in standard bioethics but closely related to it. This rather unorthodox way of dividing the book suggests that it is not necessary for the reader to start at the beginning and progress to the end. The reader can simply delve into a topic of interest since the themes that hold the topics together bind them quite loosely.

NOTES

1. Amy Harmon, "Burden of Knowledge: Tracking Prenatal Health," *New York Times*, June 20, 2004, A1, A19.

2. Warren T. Reich, ed., *The Encyclopedia of Bioethics*, 2nd ed. (New York: Simon & Schuster Macmillan, 1995). This encyclopedia is now available in a third edition, edited by Stephen Post.

3. T. Beauchamp and J. Childress, *Principles of Biomedical Ethics*, 5th ed. (New York: Oxford University Press, 2001).

4. A. Jonsen, *The Birth of Bioethics* (New York: Oxford University Press, 1997).

I

WHO LIVES? WHO DIES? WHO DECIDES? AN ESSAY ON ETHICS AND BIOETHICS

In Florida, a forty-one-year-old woman lingers for the past fifteen years of her life totally unconscious of the world around her. Her husband asks doctors to stop the life-supporting devices that provide nutrition; her parents insist that she be kept alive. The Florida courts support the husband's request, but the governor, the Florida legislature, and the Congress of the United States intervene to prevent her death. In California, the wife of former Republican president Ronald Reagan, whose mind had been ravaged by Alzheimer's disease, appeals to the Republican administration to modify its strictures on stem cell research. This form of scientific research aims to cure many diseases, but the Bush administration (which reveres President Reagan) has restricted it, considering it unethical. Stories about the Florida woman, Terri Schiavo, and about stem cell research have been staples in media coverage of bioethical issues from 2000 to 2005. I shall return to these stories later; for now, I note that both are bioethics stories: they both ask the same questions.

Who should live? Who should die? Who should decide? These are the constant questions that the field of bioethics attempts to answer. They first appeared in the headline, "They Decide Who Lives, Who Dies," for a long article in *Life* magazine in 1962.[1] That article was the first bioethical news story. It reported a new medical technique called chronic renal hemodialysis, which diverts blood from the body of a person whose kidneys have lost the ability to cleanse it of the poisons naturally accumulated in the body, passes that poisoned blood through a mechanical cleanser called an *artificial kidney*, and reinfuses it into the patient's body. People who would certainly die of kidney failure can be kept alive for years by this technique, repeated twice weekly for the rest of their lives.

This invention was hailed as a "medical miracle." It was the first genuinely life-sustaining technology. However, its inventors quickly realized that they had many more patients seeking treatment than they could accommodate. They set up a committee charged with the awesome task of choosing, from among all of the medically suitable candidates, those few who would be given dialysis. Those who were not chosen would die. A photo of the committee was spread across the two opening pages of the story: each face was shadowed, as if this anonymous committee were a panel of hanging judges or executioners. The *Life* headline was sensational but accurate.

Of course, the questions Who lives? Who dies? Who decides? have been asked since time immemorial. Rulers, generals, and judges have asked them. Tyrants distinguish those who live from those who die on the basis of their docility and servility; generals decide which troops shall spearhead the attack; judges render sentences of capital punishment on the basis of law and evidence. The *Life* article dealt, however, not with the authoritarian and punitive world of government and law but with the benign world of healing. In that world, these were new questions. Certainly, medicine has always dealt with death: its work has been to stave off death or to comfort the dying. But physicians had neither the power nor the authority to decide between life and death. They could at best distinguish in a rough way between those who seemed fated to die and those whom treatment might benefit. The answer to the ethical questions came from nature or fate, not human authority. Napoleon's army surgeons invented the rules of triage, selecting from the myriads of wounded those few whom they could save. But even these doctors could do little more than guess whether their ministrations would revive the wounded quickly enough for them to fight again. When these military "bioethicists" asked "who should live?" they were selecting wounded soldiers worth their meager efforts to save.

The modern question about life and death is different. It arises in a medical world filled with elaborate machines, extraordinary techniques, and complex drugs. These are often hailed as "medical miracles." They stop in their tracks diseases, like pneumonia and tuberculosis, that were once almost always fatal and restore patients to perfect health. They halt other diseases, such as cancer or heart disease, and hold off their fatal effects for years. Machines perform the functions of organs, such as dialysis machines for kidneys, ventilators for lungs, and pacemakers for hearts, maintaining life artificially. The three bioethical questions posed above ask about the appropriate use of this array of medical abilities. Unquestionably, these medical abilities bring great good to the sick and the dying; so, the answer to the questions Who lives? and Who dies? should be simple: all should live; no one should die. But it is not that simple, and when it is not simple, we have to ask, Who should decide?

The medical innovations and the scientific advances of the twentieth century not only revolutionized the treatment of disease; they tapped into secrets of physiology and psychology that showed how to "remake" humans. They opened the mysteries of reproduction and heredity and made it possible to "make" babies outside of the body and according to design. These possibilities seemed to bestow on scientists creative powers and, with them, the power to do both good and evil. This power recalls the tale of Frankenstein, the genius scientist who imparted life to a lifeless bundle of parts collected from cadavers. Because Frankenstein did not know how to deal with his marvelous creature, it became a monster, dangerous to all humans and to itself.

Popular writers will often refer to scientific accomplishments as "Frankensteinian." In the early days of organ transplantation, commentators sometimes compared surgeons to the mad scientist and patients to the poor, patched creature. In the early days of molecular genetics, Frankenstein lurked in the laboratories. A politician opposed Harvard's plan to build a genetics laboratory with the alarm that "Frankenstein's monsters will crawl out of the sewers of Cambridge." Opponents of genetically engineered crops call them "Frankenfoods," and genetically engineered organisms are named "Frankenbugs."

This literary reference is extravagant but pointed. The Frankenstein story, created in 1816 by Mary Wollstonecraft Shelley, is a fable of modern scientific power. The scientist, Frankenstein, has discovered the secret of life, enabling him to make dead matter alive. He also gives that living being a physical form (he intends it to be beautiful, but it turns out ugly) and a psychological character (he intends it to be benign, but his own treatment of it turns it malign). He creates it with the best of intentions—to solve the mystery of disease and death—but his good intentions go awry. Many commentators have found in this riveting novel an allegory of modern science: it has the power to create life, to sustain it, to shape its qualities; at the same time, it has not conquered death, and its mastery of nature is fallible. Bioethical questions acknowledge these powers, their limits, and above all, the responsibility that accompanies the power of creating. At the root of bioethical questions lie even more fundamental questions: what is it to be alive or, more particularly, to be alive as a human? What are the moral duties and constraints that confront us as we enhance our power over who lives and who dies (see appendix C on the Frankenstein analogy).

The word "bioethics" first appeared in print in 1969. It was invented by a medical researcher, Dr. Van Rensselaer Potter, to describe his idea of a broad field of study that would link human values with biological knowledge. The *Encyclopedia of Bioethics* defines its contents as "the systematic study of the moral dimensions—including moral vision, decisions, conduct and policies—of the life sciences and health care, employing a variety of ethical methodologies in an interdisciplinary setting."[2] The "bio" in bioethics comes from *bios*, the Greek word for life. "Life" is an elusive word, a word for poets, theologians, scientists, and for all of us who live it happily or miserably, vigorously or indolently. Life is an enigma followed by its contrary mystery, death. Scientists make it a phenomenon of organic activity, marked by empirical properties like nutrition, respiration, reproduction, and the genetic basis for these activities. Medicine seeks to comprehend its vagaries by tracing the defects in these properties. But we also use the prefix "bio" in "biography," the story of the events and experiences of an individual life. In this sense, life displays not only physical properties but also joy and tragedy, beliefs and values.

When Potter invented the word "bioethics," he saw life in its most comprehensive sense, drawing in all animate creatures and the systems that hold them together. He placed human experience within this comprehensive and evolving world. Potter hoped that the new study he envisioned would incorporate all living beings within the perspective of human values. As it happened, however, his word "bioethics" was captured by only one segment of the study of life, the biomedical sciences. Modern bioethics considers the ways in which biomedicine touches the biographies of persons. So, when bioethicists talk of life, they refer not only to the physical substratum, our chemistry, biology, and genetics, but also to conscious, social, and historical experience as we understand it, have feelings about it, and evaluate it. Bioethics, then, approaches questions about whether Terri Schiavo or a human embryo is alive, not only in the biological sense but also in the human sense, that is, as due the respect and rights recognized by morality. This is a philosophical and religious question.

ETHICS, MORAL PHILOSOPHY, AND MORAL THEOLOGY

The word "bioethics" is newly minted; the word "ethics" is old coinage. In ancient Greek, it commonly means "customs," as in the customs of the Athenian people. In his treatise *Ethics*, the philosopher Aristotle explained his views about the good life for humans. Here, the word "ethics" means more than customs; it designates the human characteristics or virtues that prepare people to live well and successfully in human communities. The word "ethics" encompasses philosophical reflection on morality and names a study that has been, for centuries, one of the major departments of philosophy. A modern *Dictionary of Philosophy* defines ethics as "the philosophical study of morality. . . . [T]he general study of goodness and the general study of right action constitute the main business of ethics. . . . Its principal substantive questions are what ends we ought, as fully rational beings, to choose and pursue and what moral principles should govern our choices and pursuits."[3]

People sometimes ask how it is possible to "study" ethics. Is not ethics a matter of personal choice and values? Must not each person form his or her own ethics? How can someone teach ethics to another person? At best, parents may direct (or push) their children into certain patterns of behavior, but once grown out of childhood, individuals must choose for themselves whether or not to accept those patterns. Ethics, it is said, cannot be taught; they can at best, say the skeptics, be "caught," like a cold.

Ethics professors have many answers to this objection (which threatens their livelihood). One answer goes this way: since ethics is about moral life, it deals with issues on which feelings often run very high and can run very wrong. Whoever attends a class on ethics or picks up a book about ethics encounters emotionally engaging questions, and as things usually go, people form their ideas about what is right or wrong and design their actions (if action is called for) under the power of their emotional response. The study of ethics should encourage people to scrutinize the reasons that might justify choice and action and to test their emotional or conventional responses against those reasons.

So, a person can study ethics if he or she is willing to consider reasonable arguments about the issues and to formulate opinions and choices in light of these arguments. This means stepping back not only from one's emotional response but also from the customs and practices that one learns as a youth or as a member of a particular community, faith, and culture. One need not reject these but should at least be willing to subject them to examination. Ethics explains the methods whereby one can examine one's preferences and choices, as well as the policies and actions of others.

People often ask whether there is a distinction between *ethics* and *morality*. The two terms can be used interchangeably since one is Greek and the other Latin for "custom." However, some philosophers will distinguish between them: morality describes the practices and conduct that arise from custom; ethics describes choices arising from reasonable examination of morality. Another way of distinguishing morality and ethics is to use "morality" to describe the actual beliefs, choices, and actions of persons and communities, reserving "ethics" for an academic activity, the philosophical study of morality. In this sense, a person can get tenure as a professor of ethics but not of morality.

The academic study of ethics mixes the words; it is often designated as "moral philosophy" or, in some religious traditions, "moral theology." Like most academic studies, these have a long tradition of reflection, issuing in libraries of books. For simplicity sake, I mark the beginning of that tradition in the fifth century BCE. During the first quarter of that century, Lord Siddartha (Buddha) of India and Kung Fu-Tse (Confucius) of China concluded long lives spent teaching humans how to live. In the second half of that same century, Socrates of Athens instructed his fellow citizens that "the unexamined life was not worth living" (*Apology*, 38a). The teachings of these almost contemporary masters initiated the disciplined reflection that has shaped moral life within their respective cultures. Our study of bioethics will remain within the Western, or Socratic, tradition of moral philosophy.

Socrates incessantly asked Athenians whether they understood the meaning of the virtues and values that they claimed to revere: he asked generals whether they knew what courage was; he asked politicians what justice meant; he asked teachers if they could define wisdom. Out of this regimen of inquiry, Socrates's followers, the moral philosophers of the Western tradition, constructed systems for seeking answers and testing their truth. One line of questioning concerned the nature of the good life for humans: Is it possible to discern ideals for life that are objectively true? Does the knowledge of these ideals make humans happy? Can humans realize ideals in their choices and actions? Are they free and responsible beings or ruled by fate? Can virtue be taught? How can humans discern the right thing to do? What is a just society? Plato, Aristotle, the Stoics and the Epicureans, Cicero, Epictetus the slave, and Marcus Aurelius the emperor reflected on these questions, examined their predecessors' answers, and formulated their own conceptions of the good life, which, they hoped, others would appreciate and approve.

The two major religious traditions that have affected Western culture, Christianity and Judaism, also contributed to these reflections. These faiths sought answers in texts that they believed to be the word of God. Yahweh imposed commandments upon his people; Jesus preached a gospel of altruistic love. The disciples who inherited these messages elaborated teachings that sometimes paralleled the philosophers' reflections and often went beyond them. St. Augustine, Thomas Aquinas, and Moses Maimonides not only reflected on the inspired words of scripture but also drew the ideas of ancient philosophy into the divine revelation. Thus, in Western culture, ethics represents broad and deep reflections on the nature and meaning of human life.

Around the time of the Enlightenment, scholars shaped these reflections into systematic theories. The ancient questions were methodically examined and set into ordered structures of thought. In England, Thomas Hobbes, John Locke, Lord Shaftsbury, Bishop Butler, David Hume, Jeremy Bentham, and John Stuart Mill, in Europe, Benedict de Spinoza, Immanuel Kant, Georg Hegel, Arthur Schopenhauer, and Friedrich Nietzsche produced masterpieces of ethical reasoning. This rich medley of ideas was siphoned into the courses on moral philosophy required in most American colleges until the mid-twentieth century. In addition to teaching, professors of philosophy devoted their intellectual skills to refining the logic of argument and the definition of terms used in ethics. This technical concern, called *metaethics*, fascinated many philosophers more than the dusty questions about the meaning of life and the determination of right action. Metaethics often marginalized these questions, and at the time when bioethics began, moral philosophy seemed an unlikely ally. (A slightly more detailed history of moral philosophy can be found in appendix A.)

So, moral philosophers and other sages ruminate endlessly about morality and the moral life. They present a great variety of views. There is no one, universally accepted moral philosophy. So, the "ethics" in bioethics does not signal that a philosophical system awaits application to the problems posed by bioscience and medicine. Rather, it suggests that out of the medley of moral philosophy, ideas can be drawn and arguments borrowed that illuminate these problems.

Among those ideas is a distinction between two quite different ways of constructing and analyzing moral arguments. Modern moral philosophy distinguishes between *deontological formalist* arguments and *consequentialist* or *utilitarian* ones. The former proposes that a moral judgment is "right" if it conforms to some rule or duty (*deon* means "duty" in Greek); the latter claims that moral judgments are justified by references to the "good" consequences that are produced by actions. A massive literature surrounds these distinctions. Philosophers refine their definitions, clarify or contest the arguments for and against them, and construct large theories to explain them. Certainly, there is much more to moral philosophy, and there are many other ways to think about moral decision making. We mention the distinction here because it frequently appears in bioethical argumentation. Curious readers can refer to the sources mentioned at the end of this essay.

Oxford moral philosopher G. J. Warnock suggests a useful way to appreciate the function of moral philosophy. He proposes that the object of moral evaluation is to contribute to the improvement (he says "amelioration") of what he calls the "human predicament." The human predicament is that "things are liable to go badly." The basic reason for this depressing fact is that humans have limited information about the world and themselves, limited intelligence to figure out what is needed, as well as when and how best to use it, and most significantly, limited sympathy; that is, they tend first to serve their own interests and those of the people they cherish. Only reluctantly do they reach out to strangers and the wider world.[4]

Warnock's view may provide a philosophical prelude to bioethics. One of the most appalling features of the human predicament is the devastation that disease and injury wreak on the human frame and on human society.

Bioethics is the ethics of biomedical science and practice, where, in general, the intentions of persons are worthy and the goals that they pursue worthwhile. Scientists seek to understand disease and to fashion cures that can be put into the hands of doctors. The betterment of the human predicament is the objective of the biomedical sciences: they aim to increase resources for the treatment and management of disease and to expand the capabilities of persons to resist and prevent disease. However, as we shall see in the following pages, this beneficent intent and objective is fraught with difficulties. Limited rationality often blocks the view of consequences; limited sympathies sometimes allow self-interest to distract from the interests of others.

Bioethics is an attempt to show how reason can be enlarged and sympathies extended as we search for the betterment of the human predicament in the world of biomedical science and medicine. Ethical arguments are crafted to illuminate the practices of science and medicine so that each achievement contributes not only to the well-being of persons (beneficence) but also enhances their autonomy (respect for persons) and promotes the fair distribution of burdens and benefits in human society (justice). And, at its essence, bioethics reflects on what it means to be alive within a scientifically understood and technologically manipulated world.

BIOETHICS

The scholarly field of bioethics started to form during the 1960s when some scientists began to converse with each other about the dangerous aspects of advances in the biomedical sciences. Physicists, particularly those involved in the development of nuclear weapons, had initiated such conversations about the social implications of their work soon after atomic bombs killed thousands at Hiroshima and Nagasaki in 1945. The astonishing, albeit less destructive, scientific advances in the biosciences were raising similar questions about their effects on human life and values. In 1962, a group of distinguished scientists gathered in London to spend three days talking at the *Man and His Future Conference*. The proceedings opened with the words, "The world was unprepared socially, politically and ethically for the advent of nuclear power. Now, biological research is in ferment, creating and promising methods of interference with 'natural processes,' which could destroy or transform nearly every aspect of human life, which we value. It is necessary for . . . every intelligent individual of our world to consider the present and imminent possibilities."[5] The discussion ranged from eugenics to mind control by drugs, from organ transplantation to antibiotics that saved lives yet led to population explosions.

The discussants were not merely critical observers; they were leading scientists who were pushing ahead the very discoveries that they were questioning.

The discussions were earnest; answers were elusive. Ethical "discussion" was little more than thoughtful, worried puzzlement: what should be done when the good things flowing from medical science seem to have bad effects? This sort of question is not, of course, a new one for humans. In every human endeavor, such as governing a society, defending a country, educating children, and making and marketing goods, efforts to succeed often entail bad consequences, and the best intentions lead to evil results. In all cultivated societies, wise persons have reflected on these problems and analyzed them in interesting ways, formulating the disciplines called ethics, moral philosophy, or, in faith traditions, moral theology. Some persons familiar with these disciplines suggested that the new problems of bioscience might profitably be exposed to the concepts and reasoning of ethics.

In 1969, a young philosopher, Daniel Callahan, founded the Institute of Society, Ethics and the Life Sciences (now the Hastings Center) to initiate intense study of the new questions. In a 1973 article, he wrote that "bioethics is not yet a full discipline. . . . [It lacks] general acceptance, disciplinary standards, criteria of excellence and clear pedagogical and evaluative norms." This very lack, he suggested, offered bioethics an unprecedented opportunity to define itself. It could move toward "definition of issues, methodological strategies and procedures for decision-making." In defining issues, bioethics would need "the rigor of the unfettered imagination," the ability to envision alternatives, to get into people's ethical agonies. In developing methodological strategies, bioethics must use the traditional modes of philosophical analysis—logic, consistency, careful use of terms, rational justification—supplemented by sensitivity to feeling and emotions as well as to political and social influences on behaviors. Finally, the discipline must provide procedures "to reach reasonably specific, clear decisions . . . in the circumstances of medicine and science."

Callahan concluded, "The discipline of bioethics should be so designed, and its practitioners so trained, that it will directly—at whatever cost to disciplinary elegance—serve those physicians and biologists whose positions demand that they make the practical decisions." This sort of discipline, according to Callahan, requires a knowledge of the sociology of the professions and of health care, scientific training, historical knowledge of philosophical theories of value, and facility both with the methods of ethical analysis common in the philosophical and theological communities and with their limitations when applied to cases—an "impossible list of demands," admitted Callahan, but approachable by "a continuing, tension-ridden dialectic . . . kept alive by a continued exposure to specific cases in all their human dimensions"[6]

At his new institute, he gathered a few philosophers, physicians, scientists, lawyers, and other scholars for occasional meetings to inaugurate the study of major issues then puzzling biomedical science and practice. A small staff of young scholars in these fields selected topics that seemed to need particular attention and organized four task forces for intense discussion. The topics chosen were death and dying, behavior control, genetic engineering, and population control. It was Callahan's belief that the complex theoretical questions that he raised in the essay quoted above would be best addressed not by private reflection in a scholar's study but by sustained, focused debate among a variety of informed persons. This approach set the style for bioethics: it has consistently relied on public discourse rather than abstract deliberation to advance understanding of its issues. Many government commissions and committees and many conferences have followed this pattern.

Theologians of the various faith traditions also joined the discussions. Many of them, such as theologian Joseph Fletcher, an Episcopalian, Princeton professor Paul Ramsey, a Methodist, and Richard McCormick, a Catholic, recognized that hidden behind the ethical problems of the laboratory and clinic were some very ancient questions: What is the meaning of life? Who has the right to live? Is it ever permissible to terminate human life? Questions like these have been the province of theologians from time immemorial. They have struggled to understand the words of scriptural revelation, which speak often about life and death, and reflected on the traditions of their communities that teach the faithful how to live and to die. Some theological traditions, such as Roman Catholicism and Judaism, also have a rich tradition of moral reflection on the practice of medicine.

Catholic, Protestant, and Jewish theologians brought to the field a resource that the philosophers did not have: substantive moral traditions about great issues of life and death. Certainly, theologians cast life in a larger, more transcendental framework than do scientists and philosophers, and when they speak of the sanctity of life, they endow it with a quality derived from a source beyond human power. Yet, the early bioethical theologians were aware that they worked in a pluralistic religious world and that their doctrines might not convince those who did not share their traditions. They frequently attempted to draw universally appealing arguments out of the heart of their traditions and to cast particular theological notions in a more secular tone.

Gradually, the theologians and the philosophers began to speak together about bioethical problems, each bringing the resources of their respective disciplines and traditions. Two years after the founding of the Hastings Center, scholarly physician André Hellegers founded the Kennedy Institute of Ethics at Georgetown University. The Kennedy Institute, like the Hastings Center, was open to philosophers and theologians alike, but it fostered the theological aspects of bioethics by engaging several leading theological scholars. One of these, Protestant theologian James Childress, teamed with another Georgetown faculty member, Tom Beauchamp, an analytically trained philosopher. They brought the theological and philosophical facets of bioethics together by coauthoring *Principles of Biomedical Ethics.* This book was the first major textbook in bioethics and remains authoritative. Its success comes not only from its clarity, comprehensiveness, and fairness; it comes as well from the conjunction of two scholarly minds, working on the same problem from diverse perspectives.

Beauchamp and Childress organize their text around four principles: respect for autonomy, nonmaleficence, beneficence, and justice. In doing so, they set the agenda for bioethics. Although many other approaches have been proposed, the Four Principle Method has achieved wide popularity. Indeed, it has been called the "Georgetown Mantra." This epithet is accurate insofar as the four principles are constantly invoked in bioethical argument; it is unfair in its implication that merely uttering them will solve complex problems. Yet, these four principles provide a base or ground for much of bioethical analysis.

The authors defined respect for autonomy as "acknowledg[ing] a person's right to hold views, to make choices, and to take actions based on personal values and beliefs." The principles of nonmaleficence and beneficence refer to the moral duty to refrain from harming persons and the obligation, under many circumstances, to contribute to their welfare. Justice refers to the complex of ideas that center around the basic moral duty to treat persons equally and fairly, in accord with their needs, efforts, contributions, and merit.[7]

Each of these principles sums up a complex set of considerations and distinctions, which the authors exactingly spell out. They then show how each principle might illuminate certain sorts of bioethical problems. These authors do not, as a moral philosopher once wrote, "think of an adult person's mind or conscience as rather like a living telephone book, stocked with moral principles of the Ten Commandment type . . . [in which] one searches for the appropriate rule or rules which then suddenly appear in our conscious thoughts"[8] Rather, they see these principles as a framework of norms within which one can reflect upon and attempt to resolve moral problems. They believe that these principles reflect "common morality," that is, principles that would be accepted by most thoughtful persons in every culture. They do not go to any great lengths to demonstrate this claim, but the Four Principles have been very widely accepted, with some modification of meaning and some additions, in international bioethics.

Beauchamp and Childress took a bold step in organizing their text around principles. When they wrote, moral philosophers were still immersed in metaethics, the logic of moral argument, and hardly favored so explicit a statement of ethical norms. Few moral philosophy texts were devoted to explication of principles as such, being more concerned about ethical theories. One of the reasons for this interest in theory was the perceived shakiness of any statement about moral principles. Undoubtedly, people appeal to principles as they think about moral questions. Thus, an author strongly tempted to slip another author's eloquent phrases into his own writing might recall a moral rule: you should not plagiarize. He might wonder why not, then remember that he was taught as a child, you should not steal, and realize that plagiarism is a form of stealing. The injunction against stealing is a moral principle, standing behind and justifying the more immediate moral rule about plagiarism.

Philosophers certainly admitted that moral reasoning worked somewhat in this way, but they would immediately point out many problems. Principles can conflict, and it is not evident which of the conflicting principles should rule. Principles are very general, and it is not obvious how they might apply to a complex situation. Above all, it is hardly clear where these principles come from: are they divine commands, imperatives of nature, cultural maxims, or summations of communal experience? With all these intellectual problems swirling around the idea of ethical principles, Beauchamp and Childress were brave to grasp certain specific principles and import them into the center of the new discipline.

As this book proceeds, we shall see how these rules and principles function in regard to the particular ethical problems under discussion. However, rules and principles do not comprehend the whole of ethics or of bioethics. Beauchamp and Childress also give an important role to moral character and to the virtues appropriate to the world of medicine: compassion, discernment, trustworthiness, integrity, and conscientiousness.

Some contemporary bioethicists judge that although Beauchamp and Childress provide a balanced array of principles, autonomy has become the dominant principle, pushing the others into the background. Physician-bioethicist Edmund Pellegrino complains that the principle of autonomy, valid as it is, overwhelms the principle of beneficence. Beneficence, he claims, is the most ancient ethical principle of medicine. Hippocrates wrote, "Be of benefit and do no harm" (*Epidemics* I, xi). This principle, suggests Pellegrino, acknowledges that sick persons are vulnerable and often suffer from severely diminished autonomy. They must be helped toward its restoration by what might otherwise be seen as paternalistic acts of healing. British philosopher Onora O'Neill has criticized bioethics' reliance on autonomy as undermining the trust that must unite physician and patient.

Other bioethicists have drawn back from debates over theory and principle to concentrate on close analysis of actual clinical cases, using a traditional method of Roman and Anglican Catholic moral theology called *casuistry* (although modern casuistry has shed its denominational robes).[9] These authors stress the facts of the case, its formal structure, and the variety of interpretations of principles that might be applicable. They search for resolutions by comparisons with similar cases. Other authors propose a *narrative ethics* in which richly described situations reveal the complexity of actors' values and motives.

Finally, two important styles of bioethics are described as *feminist* and *feminine*. These two styles are similar in that they arise from the experience of women as health care providers, caretakers, patients, and compassionate observers. They differ in that the former draws on analyses of social and cultural power to show how male hegemony defines moral issues so as to preserve male authority; the latter proposes that a style of moral perception and behavior unique to women inclines them to define moral problems more in terms of community and connectedness between people, while men define them as problems of rights and contracts. For example, feminist bioethicists may view informed consent as a mechanism of male dominance in which the flow of information from male physicians to women patients predestines the result. Women, in this view, must control the information about their own bodies. A feminine bioethics may be less skeptical about the very practice of informed consent but will approach disputes over consent to procedures not as clashes between the rights of patients and duties of doctors but as settings for negotiation and conciliation. Often feminist and feminine interpretations of the issues in this book will be striking and unique: I do not mention them often because I believe that is best done by those who speak from these points of view.

Bioethics' absorption into medicine brings it into contact with another form of ethics, namely, professional medical ethics. In every era and in all literate cultures, doctors have evoked ideals and imposed imperatives on their practice. These ideals and imperatives formed a professional ethics as healers became representatives of a learned and socially prominent body known as a *profession*. The rules of medical professional ethics aim to preserve the profession's reputation and respectability in the eyes of the public and (in the eye's of its critics) to sustain the profession's monopoly over practice. Generally, this professional ethics proposes that practitioners should maintain competence in the use of their skills and show compassion to those who come to them for help. It forbids certain acts, such as sexual contact with patients and exploitation of their vulnerability. It counsels generosity to those who cannot pay for their care. It prescribes an elaborate etiquette between practitioners (sometimes, as in the common admonition not to criticize a colleague, to the detriment of patients). These injunctions, expressed throughout the literature of medicine in the West, in China, and in India, were composed as ethical codes, with specific do's and don'ts and are commonly considered by the professions, the public, and the law as expressing the ethical duties of health care providers (see appendix B).

While philosophers might see this tradition and its codes as merely self-promoting advertising, bioethics availed itself of this traditional body of ethical norms. The principles of beneficence and nonmaleficence, for example, reflect the ancient admonition of Hippocrates: "be of benefit and do no harm." Contemporary concerns about the right to health care and the lack of access to care reflect the long tradition that even a profession that earns its living by healing must respond to those who need its help but cannot afford its prices. It is not unusual to find fragments of professional ethics appearing in the context of a bioethical argument.

So, in modern bioethics, ethics takes many forms. It resembles philosophical ethics in that it strives for clarity and accuracy in the formulation of ideas and arguments. It imports into bioethical discourse large parts of ethical theory but does not allow theory to distract from its attention to the practical. It resembles theological ethics in its concern about substantive rightness and wrongness of action, and its call for moral ideals in the world of health care. It has, however, developed its own style of practical ethics, endeavoring to formulate or criticize policies, institutions, and conduct in the light of certain principles.

In fact, that style reverts to a very ancient form of doing ethics. The Greek and Roman philosophers spoke of "inventing arguments." By "inventing," they did not mean simply making them up out of thin air. They meant that persuading or dissuading people about the right or wrong course of action required fashioning an argument out of the facts of the situation, a variety of moral considerations, and some commonplace truths about human behavior. That argument should be designed to fit the question. This "invention" of arguments is somewhat like a pianist's improvisation in a classical concerto. The invention of arguments in practical ethics is an improvisation because, like the classical soloist, the ethicist must improvise by starting with themes already laid down. Ethical improvisation consists of the movement of mind seeking to understand concepts and arguments as they appear in particular issues and cases. It relates general themes to events in time, institutional structures, cultural conventions, professional practices, and many other features of the world of personal and social experience.

Thus, the ethics of bioethics is not a clean, closed system of rational argument. No theory dominates bioethics, and no methodology has won universal acceptance. While a few bioethicists, such as Princeton professor Peter Singer, adhere to such a system (in his case, to a strictly logical utilitarianism), most bioethicist today are improvisers, drawing from various forms of philosophical and theological ethics the elements that seem suitable for the argument at hand. The themes of respect for autonomy, nonmaleficence, beneficence, and justice, so well articulated by Beauchamp and Childress, are constantly invoked in the improvisation, but many other approaches are employed as well. Beauchamp favors a consequentialist form of ethical argument; Childress prefers the deontological style. Like them, most bioethicists can be utilitarians or deontologists as the occasion demands. Virtues, such as compassion or fidelity, are also constants of the discussion. This eclectic approach to ethics distresses those academic philosophers who insist that ethics must be an univocal system of logical argument. Nevertheless, it has served well to illuminate and inform the discourse about bioethical issues when they arise in the clinic, laboratory, and forums of public policy.

A word must be said about the link between bioethics and the law. Law deals with life and death in the most concrete way: it seeks out and punishes murderers, it prohibits endangering life and limb, it regulates medical practice, it limits abortion. Over the centuries, it has developed legal theories that encompass these and many other aspects of life and health. It has adjudicated cases and passed statutes about them. Inevitably, the questions of bioethics mingle with the questions of the law. From the beginning of bioethics, legal scholars have joined the discussion. Many cases involving bioethical questions have come to the courts. Legislatures have passed laws that reflect various bioethical positions. So, it is impossible to describe the field of bioethics without reference to "biolaw," and the reader will find many references in the following pages. Despite the prominence of law, a bioethics that seeks to alleviate the human predicament must be, in essence, a philosophical and theological enterprise.

NOTES

1. S. Alexander, "They Decide Who Lives, Who Dies," *Life* 53 (1962): 102–25.

2. W. Reich, ed., *Encylopedia of Bioethics*, Vol. 1, rev. ed. (New York: Simon & Schuster Macmillan, 1995), xxi.

3. R. Audi, ed., *The Cambridge Dictionary of Philosophy* (Cambridge: Cambridge University Press, 1999), 284.

4. G. J. Warnock, *The Object of Morality* (London: Methuen, 1971), 26.

5. G. Wolstenholme, *Man and His Future* (Boston: Little, Brown and Co., 1963), 2.

6. D. Callahan, "Bioethics as a Discipline," *Hastings Center Studies* 1 (1973): 66–73.

7. T. Beauchamp and J. Childress, *Principles of Biomedical Ethics*, 5th ed. (New York: Oxford University Press, 2001), 63, 114, 166, 226.

8. R. Brandt, *Ethical Theory* (Englewood Cliffs, NJ: Prentice Hall, 1959), 246.
9. A. R. Jonsen and S. E. Toulmin, *The Abuse of Casuistry: A History of Moral Reasoning* (Berkeley: University of California Press, 1987).

BIBLIOGRAPHY

Annas, G. 2005. *American Bioethics: Crossing Human Rights and Health Law Boundaries.* New York: Oxford University Press.
Beauchamp, T., and J. Childress. 2001. *Principles of Biomedical Ethics.* New York: Oxford University Press.
Blackburn, S. 2000. *Being Good.* New York: Oxford University Press.
Campbell, A., G. Gillett, and G. Jones. 2001. *Medical Ethics.* New York: Oxford University Press.
Dorff, E. 1993. *Matters of Life and Death: A Jewish Approach to Modern Medical Ethics.* Philadelphia: Jewish Publishing Society.
Engelhardt, H. 1986. *The Foundations of Bioethics.* New York: Oxford University Press.
Fiore, R., and H. L. Nelson, eds. 2003. *Recognition, Responsibility and Rights: Feminist Ethics and Social Theory.* Lanham, MD: Rowman & Littlefield.
Fletcher, Jos. 1954. *Morals and Medicine: The Moral Problems of the Patient's Right to Know the Truth, Contraception, Artificial Insemination, Sterilization and Euthanasia.* Princeton, NJ: Princeton University Press.
Gillon, R. 1994. *Principles of Health Care Ethics.* Chichester: John Wiley & Sons.
Harris, J. 2001. *Bioethics.* New York: Oxford University Press.
Jonsen, A. 1998. *The Birth of Bioethics.* New York: Oxford University Press.
Jonsen, A. 2001. *A Short History of Medical Ethics.* New York: Oxford University Press.
Mackler, A. 2003. *Introduction to Jewish and Catholic Bioethics.* Washington, DC: Georgetown University Press.
McCormick, R. 1981. *How Brave a New World: Dilemmas in Bioethics.* Garden City, NY: Doubleday.
Menikoff, J. 2001. *Law and Bioethics: An Introduction.* Washington, DC: Georgetown University Press.
Nelson, J. L. 2002. *Hippocrates' Maze: The Ethical Exploration of the Medical Labyrinth.* Lanham, MD: Rowman & Littlefield.
Pellegrino, E., and D. Thomasma. 1981. *For the Patient's Good: The Restoration of Beneficence in Health Care.* New York: Oxford University Press.
Post, Stephen, ed. 2003. *Encyclopedia of Bioethics*, 3rd. ed. New York: Macmillan.
Ramsey, P. 2002. *The Patient as Person: Explorations in Medical Ethics*, 2nd ed. New Haven, CT: Yale University Press.
Reich, W., ed. 1997. *Encyclopedia of Bioethics*, 2nd ed. New York: Macmillan.
Rothman, D. 1991. *Strangers at the Bedside: A History of How Law and Bioethics Transformed Medical Decision Making.* New York: Basic Books.
Singer, P., and H. Kuhse. 1998. *Bioethics: An Anthology.* Oxford: Blackwell.

Steinbock, B., J. Arras, and A. London. 2003. *Ethical Issues in Modern Medicine*, 6th ed. New York: McGraw-Hill.

TenHaave, H. 2001. *Bioethics in European Perspective*. Dordrecht: Kluwer Academic Publishing.

Timmons, M. 2002. *Moral Theory. An Introduction*. Lanham, MD: Rowman & Littlefield.

Veatch, R. M. 1981. *A Theory of Medical Ethics*. New York: Basic Books.

Verhay, A., and S. Lammers, eds. 1993. *Theological Voices in Medical Ethics*. Grand Rapids, MI.: Eerdmans.

Wolf, S. 1996. *Feminism and Bioethics: Beyond Reproduction*. New York: Oxford University Press.

Journals

American Journal of Bioethics (online). University of Pennsylvania Center for Bioethics, at www.bioethics.upenn.edu.

Cambridge Quarterly of Healthcare Ethics. Cambridge University Press, at www.journals.cup.org.

Hastings Center Report. The Hastings Center, 21 Malcolm Gordon Road, Garrison, New York, 10524-5555.

Journal of Clinical Ethics. 17100 Cole Road, Suite 312, Hagerstown, MD, 21740, at www.clinicalethics.com.

Journal of Medical Ethics. Institute of Medical Ethics (UK), BMJ Bookshop, Tavistock Square, London, United Kingdom, WC1H9JP, at www.bmjbookshop.com.

Medicine, Health Care and Philosophy. European Society for Philosophy of Medicine and Health Care, Kluwer Academic Publishers, P.O. Box 358, Accord Station, Hingham, MA, 02018-0358.

Theoretical Medicine and Bioethics. Springer Science and Business Media. www.springeronline.org.

II

CLINICAL BIOETHICS

$\mathcal{P}$art II is devoted to clinical bioethics. The topics discussed under this heading are those ethical problems that arise in the clinical setting, that is, when a physician is caring for a patient. The questions Who lives? Who dies? Who decides? are often straightforward; the answers are determined by the facts of the case. However, these facts can be complicated and difficult. The complexity arises when it is not clear what course of action or outcome is beneficial for the patient. Complexity is also introduced when it is not possible to know what the patient wants or when the patient's wishes do not appear beneficial. So, the broad bioethical principles of beneficence and autonomy must be fitted to particular situations. The following topics review seven areas where clinical bioethics finds ample material for serious reflection: the definition of death, forgoing life support, the autonomy of patients, euthanasia, organ transplantation, assisted reproduction, and abortion.

Defining Death

"Brain Dead Woman Dies after Fifteen Years"

$\mathcal{I}$n December 1990, a twenty-six-year-old married woman, Terri Schiavo, suffered cardiac arrest, followed by severe deprivation of oxygen to her brain. She remained in a coma for several weeks, then passed into a condition that neurological consultants designated "persistent vegetative state" (PVS)—that is, biologically alive but totally and permanently uncommunicative and unresponsive to her surroundings. She remained in that condition for fifteen years. During those years, she was required to receive nutrients and water through a tube inserted into her stomach. She was able to breathe on her own and so did not require ventilator support. Several years into her condition, her husband, Michael Schiavo, was appointed her legal guardian. Michael won a $1 million malpractice suit against the hospital into which she was first admitted. This money was used to pay for supportive care but Michael would be permitted to inherit any remainder of that sum at her death. Michael studied nursing in order to care for Terri. Some years after Terri's tragedy, Michael met another woman, with whom he is now living. The two of them have had two children. In May 1998, Michael petitioned the court to have Terri's nutrition discontinued. He testified that Terri had told him that she would not want life support, although there is no documentation to that effect. After two court reviews, Michael Schiavo's petition was granted.

After the court authorized an end to tube feeding, Terri's parents contested the court's decision. They claimed that Michael had abused their daughter; further, they intimated that Michael had caused the injuries leading to her current condition and stated that they knew that their daughter was contemplating a divorce. Terri's parents also claimed that her neurological diagnosis was mistaken and that Terri was able to communicate to them. After failing to obtain court support, Terri's parents requested that Florida governor Jeb Bush intervene on their behalf. At the governor's behest, the Florida legislature passed "Terri's Law," a special statute authorizing the governor to issue a "one time stay to prevent the withholding of nutrition and hydration." The tube, which had been withdrawn on October 15, 2003, was reinserted six days later on Governor Bush's orders. Michael Schiavo then petitioned the Florida Court of Appeals to overturn the governor's stay as an unconstitutional violation of the separation of judicial and executive branches, while the state moved to dismiss that suit. The Florida Supreme Court judged that "Terri's Law" was unconstitutional and the tube was again removed, then reinserted pending further appeal. In March 2005, the U.S. Congress passed legislation permitting Terri's case to be heard in federal jurisdictions; all federal courts, including the U.S. Supreme Court, however, refused to hear the case. Terri died on March 31, 2005.

A furious debate over Terri's fate engaged not only her family but lawyers and judges, news commentators and columnists, priests and preachers, legislators, a governor and a president, and the wider public, some of whom held vigils and demonstrations. Bioethicists were quoted on all aspects of the case. The questions raised about Terri were questions that echoed the very beginnings of the field of bioethics. Not only did the early bioethicists ask who should live or die, they also asked a more fundamental question: what is death? By the time Terri Schiavo's case came on the scene, it was understood by doctors, bioethicists, and many people that Terri was not dead. She existed in what neurologists describe as a PVS. Yet many people feel that this form of existence, totally cut off from human communication and lacking even self-consciousness, is "as good as dead." Indeed, in many opinion surveys, most respondents (more than 80 percent) considered PVS a state "worse than death."

Yet it has not always been obvious that death and PVS should be considered distinct. One of the first questions to instigate bioethical reflection was "how should death be defined?" This topic will examine that question. In topic two, I will pursue the question further: what is the ethical approach to patients in PVS, like Terri Schiavo?

DEFINING DEATH

Humans have always recognized death: a moving, speaking person becomes motionless and silent, eyes become vacant and unseeing, breathing ceases, and putrefaction sets in. At this point, the family begins to mourn. Religious rituals are performed, and the body is prepared for disposition. Although the physiology of death itself remains obscure, the last breath is a compelling sign. Myth, religion, common sense, and common law have enshrined that moment as the end of life. In many languages, "breath" and "spirit" share the same word, and in many cultures and religions, the last breath marks the departure of the person's spirit from the body it had animated. Jewish law from ancient times has respected that sign: Moses Maimonides wrote, "If, upon examination, no sign of breathing can be detected at the nose . . . he is already dead."[1]

Death has long concerned civil and criminal law since the cause of death and when it occurs can have momentous legal consequences. Law has directed doctors to declare death according to their best knowledge. Throughout history, that best knowledge was the simple observation of the signs that every person could recognize. In the sixteenth century, medical science began to appreciate the relation between respiration and circulation of the blood. Whatever the cause, failure of the lungs to deliver oxygen to the blood leads rapidly to unconsciousness and death. *Black's Law Dictionary* defines death as "the cessation of life . . . defined by physicians as a total stoppage of the circulation of the blood and a cessation of the animal and vital functions consequent thereon, such as respiration, pulsation, etc." This formula is called the cardiorespiratory (heartbeat and breathing) definition of death.

By the mid-twentieth century, the ventilator, a newly developed mechanical support for breathing, could sustain that function and, through it, other vital functions. Some persons could survive serious events, such as strokes and heart attacks, yet fail to recover consciousness; dependant on medical technology such as ventilation and dialysis, they were lost to the world of sensation and communication, living in every way except in their consciousness. Questions arose as to the appropriate treatment of such persons? Should they be considered dead? Should the medical technology that sustained organic functions, such as respiration and nutrition, be stopped? A second question also became urgent. The new technique of transplanting organs from one person to another also required a clear definition of death: kidneys and hearts must be removed from persons sufficiently "alive" that the organs are viable for transplantation but "dead" enough that the removal of the organs is not a criminal assault on the patient's life. Much confusion attended these questions.

When ventilator support and transplantation entered medical practice, neurologists were studying electrical activity in the brains of patients who were in profound coma. They correlated the absence of electrical activity in the brain with irreversible failure of that organ. It was suggested that this condition constituted a sort of death of the brain, diagnosable by technical means, with a reliable prognosis that consciousness would never return. This research suggested that a new way of determining death could be added to, or could substitute for, the cardiorespiratory signs that had traditionally been used. But was brain death equivalent to the death of the person?

The medical literature manifested uncertainty: persons who were the sources of organs were described variously as "dead" or "immanently dead" or "irreversibly dying." Problematic legal cases arose. In England, organs were taken from Mr. Potter who, to the transplanter, was "virtually dead" but, to the coroner, was still alive. In America, Clarence Nicks was beaten "to death" by an assailant, but after he was placed on a respirator, his heart continued to beat until it was transplanted into John Stuckwish. The prosecutor worried that an indictment against Mr. Nick's assailant would be clouded by the surgeon's action. The defendant's attorney said, "It will be our contention that Nicks wasn't dead." In Japan, a surgeon removed a heart from a drowned man who, in the view of other physicians, could have been resuscitated. This event aroused a public antipathy among the Japanese toward brain death and heart transplantation that has taken years to overcome.

In 1968, a committee of the Harvard University Medical School attempted to dispel the uncertainty. They published "A Definition of Irreversible Coma: Report of the Ad Hoc Committee at Harvard Medical School to Examine the Definition of Brain Death."[2] The report recognized that a new definition of death is needed for two reasons: "(1) improvements in resuscitative and supportive measures have led to increased efforts to save those who are desperately injured. Sometimes these efforts have led to partial success so that the result is an individual whose heart continues to beat but whose brain is irreversibly damaged . . . (2) obsolete criteria for definition of death can lead to controversy in obtaining organs for transplantation." The report stated the physical and neurological characteristics of irreversible coma: unresponsiveness, no movements or breathing, no reflexes, and "of great confirmatory value, a flat electroencephalogram."

The report became authoritative soon after its publication. It canonized the concept of brain death, gave physicians guidance in diagnosing that condition, and gave transplanters access to fresh organs. Prosecutors could avoid the embarrassing situation of indicting transplant surgeons as murderers. States could more easily justify statutes that recognized these new criteria. By the end of the decade, twenty-seven states had passed laws recognizing brain death. Two other organizations published statements in 1968 with nearly the same criteria for brain death—one from the French Ministry of Health and the other from the Council for International Organizations of Medical Sciences.

Despite this progress in understanding and in legislation, uncertainty remained about brain death. The scientific basis of the Harvard report and its formulations did not satisfy some observant readers. The difference between permanent unconsciousness, usually caused by cerebral damage and to which the term *brain death* was often applied, and a state of total organic disintegration perplexed physicians and the public. Indeed, the Harvard report added to the confusion by its title, "Definition of Irreversible Coma."

The term *irreversible coma* properly applies to the condition called PVS and describes a condition like Terri Schiavo's, in which the patient suffers major damage to the cerebral cortex, the part of the brain where sensation and thinking are mediated. If this damage is so severe as to be irreversible, the person is "lost to the world." The body continues metabolic and physiological activities, retains reflex responses, such as withdrawal from painful stimuli, and goes through sleep-wake cycles. Eyes sometimes seem to track light or movement. The patient will groan, yawn, even seem to weep. Many observers are convinced that these activities reveal consciousness. However, systematic evaluation demonstrates that these patients are not performing any meaningful behaviors. They cannot comprehend, cannot communicate and, indeed, lack sensation and reflective consciousness. Brain imaging and autopsies show significant destruction of those parts of the brain that make these activities possible. If this state continues for a prolonged period (more than three months for damage caused by loss of oxygen and more than a year for patients whose brains have been physically injured, as in an automobile accident), the state is called "persistent" or "permanent." These patients are highly unlikely ever to improve and, if they do, the improvement is slight, leaving the patient severely mentally and physically damaged.

The term "brain death"—used interchangeably with "irreversible coma" in the Harvard report—confuses two quite distinct physical states. In one, as the report states, "function is abolished at cerebral, brain stem, and often spinal levels." When this happens, lungs and other major organs will stop functioning, leading to organic deterioration. In fact, the Harvard report states the neurological signs that detect such total abolition of function. In the other state, function is abolished only at the cerebral level, where consciousness is generated. A human in the first state simply ceases all living activities and is, in the usual sense, dead; a person in the second state loses all conscious activities but remains alive. The confusion is fostered by common and professional language. The public constantly describes persons who have tragically lost consciousness permanently as brain dead. Doctors constantly describe persons whose loss of all organic function is detected by neurological signs while they continue to breath on a respirator as brain dead. Both are confused. While persons in PVS do not have the electrochemical and physiological activities that give brains the power of consciousness, the term "brain dead" implies, incorrectly, that the patient is dead. While patients on a respirator may be declared dead because neurological signs show that their entire organism has lost its vitality, even though they continue to breath, they are fully dead. More properly, it should be said that they are "dead as diagnosed by brain criteria." Thus, the headline that opens this topic, "Brain Dead Woman Dies after Fifteen Years" is confused and confusing. Confusion is an invitation to philosophers.

THE ETHICAL ARGUMENTS

Prof. Hans Jonas was the first philosopher to speak on this topic. While he agreed with the Harvard report's first rationale for the redefinition of death, namely, allowing permanently unconscious patients to die, he strongly disagreed with the second rationale, namely, the designation of a permanently unconscious person as dead for the purpose of removing organs for transplant. In an article entitled "Against the Stream," Jonas stood against the torrent of efforts to redefine death so that the human organism, once it lost all higher functions, could be mined for organs and, in the long run, become a thing of which any socially beneficial use could be made. He said,

> We must remember that what the Harvard group offered was not a definition of irreversible coma as a rationale for breaking off sustaining action, but a definition of death by the criterion of irreversible coma as a rationale for transposing the patient's body to the class of dead things, regardless of whether sustaining action is kept up or broken off. . . . [This was] motivated not by the exclusive interests of the patient but with extraneous interests in mind. . . . [Thus,] they serve the ruling pragmatism of our time which will let no ancient fear and trembling interfere with the relentless expanding of the realm of sheer thinghood and unrestricted utility.[3]

It is obvious that Jonas read the Harvard report as a statement about permanent unconsciousness rather than total organic deterioration. Bioethicist Robert Veatch was also a vocal critic of the Harvard criteria. He wrote that although the report stated that its primary purpose was to define irreversible coma as a new criterion of death, it never provided an argument that irreversible coma was synonymous with the death of the person as a whole. The report, Veatch correctly recognized, was a statement of technical criteria to predict the irreversibility of prolonged coma. But, he wondered, should persons in irreversible coma be treated as if they are dead? A person should be considered dead, he stipulated, when a complete loss of some essential characteristic justifies a radical change in status. Veatch suggested four different concepts of death that might make this general stipulation more specific: irreversible loss of the soul, irreversible stopping of "vital" body fluids, irreversible loss of bodily integration, and irreversible loss of consciousness or capacity for species interaction. Each of these concepts of death has been widely accepted at various times in various places; each represents a different view of what constitutes the essential characteristics of a person. The Harvard report failed to address any of these issues.[4]

Sufficient doubt, confusion, and concern persisted during the decade after the Harvard report that the U.S. Congress ordered the Presidential Commission on the Study of Ethical Problems in Medicine to study "the ethical and legal implications of the matter of defining death, including the advisability of developing a uniform definition of death." In its report, *Defining Death* (1981), the commission suggested statutory legislation that would define death as follows:

> An individual who has sustained either (1) irreversible cessation of circulatory and respiratory functions, or (2) irreversible cessation of all functions of the entire brain, including the brain stem, is dead. A determination of death must be made in accordance with accepted medical standards.[5]

This formulation expressed the commission's conclusion that death was a unitary phenomenon that can be demonstrated either on the traditional grounds of irreversible cessation of heart and lung function or on the basis of irreversible loss of all functions of the entire brain. Its definition rested on the scientific claims that the brain stem provided the physiological mechanism for the integration and unity of the living body. Once brain stem function is lost, the integrity of the organism as a whole is lost.

The commissioners had heard some philosophers claiming that a "higher brain" definition was theoretically more convincing: death should be counted from the time of an irreversible loss of personality and the attendant functions of cognition and choice. In this view, a person in PVS should be counted as dead. The commissioners, however, judged that such a definition would be too radical: it would classify as "dead" a multitude of breathing persons whose organic functions were intact, either precipitating their disposal or opening their bodies to the pragmatic purposes that had troubled Jonas. It could sweep, at least in theory, persons with profound dementia or retardation into the category of cadavers. Thus, the Uniform Definition of Death Act was accepted by most states, and the "whole-brain" definition of death has become the standard in the United States and in most of the world.

Still, many problems remain. The first is the theoretical question posed by philosophers and raised by many sensitive persons: should we decide that certain states of human existence are "worse than death," in particular, the loss of all ability to engage in human interaction as in PVS. Is it right simply to declare PVS patients dead since they are certainly "dead to the world"? Also, although the neurological profession generally supports the new definition, some scientists continue to question the assertion that the brain stem acts as the integrative organ for the living body, noting that certain physiological functions survive even total brain death. The problem of determining death that preexisted bioethics has persisted through long debates and detailed legislation. Much has been clarified, but much remains open to serious moral reflection. That reflection must go deeper than the principles of bioethics: it must penetrate to the nature of the human person.

Thus, the bioethical discussion made it clear that Terri Schiavo was not dead as defined by the criteria for whole-brain death. She was alive; discontinuing nutrients would cause her to die. The PVS deprived her of the significant human qualities of reflective thought, communication, and experience. Now the question can be asked more precisely: is the loss of these qualities so bad that it absolves others from the usual moral obligation to preserve her life by medical means? Was Terri's life of such poor quality that no one had a duty to sustain it? Was the benefit of life no longer beneficial to Terri Schiavo? Terri's sad story is not the first that raised this question. At the very beginning of bioethics, another young woman, Karen Ann Quinlan, forced the nation, its legal authorities, its medical providers, and its religious leaders to meditate on the question. We shall hear her story in the next topic.

NOTES

1. Moses Maimonides, "Hilchot Shabbat," *Mishnah Torah* 2.19.
2. "A Definition of Irreversible Coma: Report of the Ad Hoc Committee at Harvard Medical School to Examine the Definition of Brain Death," *Journal of the American Medical Association* 205 (1968): 337–40.
3. H. Jonas, "Against the Stream," *Philosophical Essays. From Ancient Creed to Technological Man* (Englewood Cliffs, NJ: Prentice Hall, 1974), 138, 140.
4. R. Veatch, *Death, Dying and the Biological Revolution: Our Last Quest for Responsibility* (New Haven, CT: Yale University Press, 1976), ch. 1.
5. President's Commission for the Study of Ethical Problems in Medicine, "Defining Death," in *Source Book in Bioethics*, ed. A. Jonsen, R. Veatch, and L. Walters (Washington, DC: Georgetown University Press, 1998), 118–42.

BIBLIOGRAPHY

Nuland, S. 1993. *How We Die*. New York: Knopf.

Potts, M., P. Byrne, and R. Nilges, eds. *Beyond Brain Death: The Case against Brain Based Criteria for Human Death*. Dordrecht, Netherlands: Kluwer Academic Publishers.

President's Commission for the Study of Ethical Problems in Medicine. 1998 [1981]. *Defining Death: Medical, Legal and Ethical Issues*. In *Source Book in Bioethics*, ed. A. Jonsen, R. Veatch, and L. Walters, 118–42. Washington, DC: Georgetown University Press.

Reich, W. 1995. "Death, Definition and Determination of," *Encyclopedia of Bioethics*. New York: Macmillan.

Russell, T. 2000. *Brain Death: Philosophical Concepts and Problems*. Aldershot, UK: Ashgate Publishing.

Youngner, S., R. Arnold, and R. Schapiro, eds. 1999. *The Definition of Death: Contemporary Controversies*. Baltimore: Johns Hopkins University Press.

Zaner, R., ed. 1988. *Death: Beyond the Whole-Brain Criteria*. Dordrecht, Netherlands: Kluwer Academic Publishers.

• *Topic 2* •

Forgoing Life Support:
The Quality of Life

"Quinlan's Life Support Removed"

$\mathcal{K}$aren Ann Quinlan, age twenty-one, was rushed to the emergency department of a small New Jersey hospital. She was unconscious, with very shallow breathing. The cause of her coma, as could best be determined, was ingestion of valium and alcohol. Doctors put her on a respirator to support her breathing. She was transferred to a larger hospital where, after a five-month stay, she was still dependent on the respirator. Her neurological condition deteriorated to what neurologists described as persistent vegetative state (PVS). Her parents requested that the doctor stop the respirator. He refused, saying this violated his medical duty. The hospital backed up his refusal, fearing that Karen's death might lead to homicide charges. The Quinlan family sought spiritual guidance from their Catholic bishop, who stated that church teaching allowed removal of "extraordinary means" of life support. The Quinlans, relieved in conscience, then sought legal relief in the New Jersey courts. The Supreme Court of the state upheld Mr. Quinlan's guardianship, and he terminated respiratory support. Karen began to breath spontaneously. She lived another nine years, never regaining consciousness.

The drama of Karen Ann Quinlan was played in the media during 1975 and 1976. Her high school graduation picture became familiar to millions. Her case was the first of its kind to reach an American court. Bioethics grew up around her story, providing concepts and arguments. It was clear from the beginning that Karen was not dead, according to the brain-death criteria. She was living in PVS, breathing only with the aid of a respirator, nourished only through a tube implanted in her chest. It was the quality of her life that was at issue: was she living a life of such low quality that her parents and providers were not obliged to support it?

The new profession of bioethicists participated in the national debate. One of its leaders, Robert Veatch, advised the Quinlan's lawyers. The New Jersey Supreme Court issued an eloquent opinion that quoted the nascent bioethical literature and, in turn, made its mark on bioethics. Although the judges' decision turned on the legal points concerning Mr. Quinlan's guardianship and the criteria for a surrogate decision, their opinion contained language that placed the quality of Karen's life at the center of ethical reflection.

> We have no doubt, in these unhappy circumstances, that if Karen were herself miraculously lucid for an interval (not altering the existing prognosis of the condition to which she would soon return) and perceptive of her irreversible condition, she could effectively decide upon discontinuance of the life-support apparatus, even if it meant the prospect of a natural death. . . . We have no hesitancy in deciding . . . that no external compelling interest of the State could compel Karen to endure the unendurable, only to vegetate a few measurable months with no realistic possibility of returning to any semblance of cognitive or sapient life.[1]

This passage is rhetorical and counterfactual: Karen could not come back and see herself in her unconscious state; she could not endure the unendurable because she could not experience at all. Still, the judicial argument is poignantly compelling. Perhaps it is a mistake even to speak of quality of life when the person has no experience of any sort of quality. The President's Commission on the Study of Ethical Problems in Medicine takes this tack when it writes about cases like Karen's:

> Treatment ordinarily aims to benefit a patient through preserving life, relieving pain and suffering, protecting against disability and returning maximally effective functioning. If a prognosis of permanent unconsciousness is correct, however, continued treatment cannot confer such benefits. Pain and suffering are absent, as are joy, satisfaction, and pleasure. Disability is total and no return to even a minimal level of social or human functioning is possible.[2]

The commission does concede that prognosis may be erroneous. Since "persistence" has to be predicted on the basis of the records of past patients in this condition, every new case poses the possibility that recovery to some form of "cognitive, sapient life" will occur. However, in light of wide experience, this possibility is vanishingly small. Among the thousands of patients in this condition, a handful are known to have "awakened"; all of these remained profoundly damaged. Terri Schiavo's parents banked on their daughter winning the unlikely bet of recovery. Karen Ann's parents looked at her with no such hope. The commission's comment admits that the only interest that such a patient could have is this slight probability of recovery: otherwise the patient has no "interests" at all.

This is an important point: our question is not exactly, Should Terri or Karen die? More exactly, are those responsible for their care and those concerned about them morally obliged to perform the actions that preserve their lives—in Karen's case, continuing respiratory support; in Terri's, continuing to give her artificial nutrients, water, and, when necessary, antibiotics for infections or putting her on a respirator or on dialysis? More precisely, the question becomes, What interests of the patient do these actions serve? As the commission suggests, they serve no interests because these patients are now and will always be incapable of appreciating any state of their existence. Thus, it can be concluded, no medical support is obligatory.

In other words, medical support is "futile." A large bioethical dispute has raged around this little word. Futile literally means incapable of producing the intended effect (it comes from a Latin word meaning "leaky," as in leaky bucket). Certainly, medical technology can usually produce its intended effect: a respirator can effect the gas exchange necessary to keep oxygen in the blood and tissues; a carefully concocted mix of nutrients delivered into the blood stream by a tube will sustain metabolism indefinitely. But the intended effect of medical technology goes beyond physical effects: it aims at the repelling of disease and the restoration of health. In medicine, futility can mean both the very low probability that this effect will be achieved, or it can refer to the quality of life attained if the effect is achieved. In these cases, and others like them, futility carries both meanings. It is a maxim of medical ethics that interventions, once they are seen to be futile, are no longer obligatory. The problem is knowing when treatment reaches this point.

The debate over futility also arose in another situation that frequently occurs in clinical medicine. The procedure called cardiopulmonary resuscitation revives a heart that has suddenly stopped by an aggressive combination of chest massage, forced mouth-to-mouth breathing, electric shock to the heart, and heart-stimulating drugs. After it was introduced in the 1950s, it was widely used both in hospitals and by emergency responders. However, it was noticed that in many persons, this strenuous intervention failed, and those that survived soon died of the underlying diseases that had brought on their cardiac arrest. Providers began to ask whether it was possible to determine when cardiac resuscitation might be futile and thus omitted. Today, it is common to designate seriously ill, hospitalized patients as "Do not resuscitate" with their own or their family's permission, when doctors judge that resuscitation would be futile, that is, would not serve the patient's interests.

Karen Ann Quinlan's parents and the judges agreed that she would have judged ventilator support futile, for it supported life without quality. Terri Schiavo's husband felt the same about the artificial nutrition that kept her alive. Yet some would insist that there is a major moral distinction between ventilator and artificial nutrition. The former supports functions (brain or lung) so damaged that, once support is removed, life ends. Turning off the respirator allows death to occur. Artificial nutrition, on the other hand, simply provides the food and water needed by any living organism: to stop feeding causes death. Philosophers and theologians argue over this distinction yet the majority condone discontinuing nutrition, seeing it as a medical procedure not unlike artificial ventilation. This was even the opinion of most Catholic theologians, although in 2004 Pope John Paul II asserted that artificial nutrition was an ordinary means of care and thus obligatory even for patients in PVS (Catholic theologians debate the meaning and force of this papal statement). Also, many people find the idea of starving a patient repugnant and unethical. However, the concept of starvation, attending with the pangs of hunger, is certainly not applicable to persons in PVS, who have no sensations or consciousness.

An important point about this argument over refraining from lifesaving treatment must be noted. It could be said that the whole argument is going wrong. Obligations do not arise because interests are served; nor are they contingent on the quality of life attained. Obligations arise because life itself is sacred. Some assert this because their religious faith dictates it; others see it as the obvious first premise of all ethical values. The sanctity of life can, and probably should be, a broad principle, whether taken as divine command or moral concept. However, broad principles rarely cover all situations. Even those faith communities, such as Judaism and Catholicism, that extol the sanctity of life as divine command allow for exceptions: killing in defense of self or dependants or country. These faiths also allow for degrees of effort in preserving life, particularly in terminal illness. Thus, it is possible to honor the sanctity of life and, at the same time, make room for forgoing life support under certain circumstances.

Another objection must be met. If life without quality or interests need not be preserved, what are we to say about those tragic humans who, from birth or by accident, have no communication with the world. Do these lives have no value? Should they be ignored or, in the extreme, eliminated? The argument about the medical support of persons in PVS may seem to teeter on the edge of the slippery slope that slides into disdain for and the destruction of many other human beings (indeed, some might say that such persons are not "human"). But ethical arguments must be carefully cut to fit the moral problem faced: arguments cut too broadly cover over quite different situations. Here the question is not, Are persons in PVS and profoundly mentally disabled individuals worthwhile? It is, Should persons now in PVS, due to trauma of one sort or another, be kept alive by medical technology? The same question can be asked about a severely retarded person if and when that person contracts a serious illness requiring life support, but it must be asked in terms of the specific quality of life of that person at that time, not in terms of his or her congenital condition.

The case of Karen Ann Quinlan was resolved in the supreme court of her state, New Jersey. That court determined that her father should be her guardian and that he could order that supportive care be terminated. The case of Terri Schiavo moved through the courts of Florida. Every court recognized that much law existed about similar cases and that, indeed, the U.S. Supreme Court had ruled on a similar case. In 1990, it concluded in the similar case of Nancy Cruzan that "a State may apply a clear and convincing evidence standard in proceedings where a guardian seeks to discontinue nutrition and hydration of a person in persistent vegetative state." Justice John Paul Stevens summarized, "This case is the first in which we consider whether, and how, the Constitution protects the liberty of seriously ill persons to be free from life-sustaining medical treatment."[3] Despite the consistent permission of Florida courts, Terri continued to live because we have not yet addressed the last of the bioethical questions: who decides? The Supreme Court speaks of the "guardian" who seeks to discontinue support. Terri's husband was appointed her guardian; her parents contested that appointment. Governor Bush assumed responsibility with the authority of the legislature. The U.S. Congress intervened. Who should decide? Our next topic explores that question.

NOTES

1. Supreme Court of New Jersey, "In the Matter of Karen Ann Quinlan" (1976), in *Source Book in Bioethics*, ed. A. Jonsen, R. Veatch, and L. Walters (Washington, DC: Georgetown University Press), 146.

2. President's Commission for the Study of Ethical Problems in Medicine, "Deciding to Forego Life-Sustaining Treatment" (1983), in *Source Book in Bioethics*, ed. A. Jonsen, R. Veatch, and L. Walters, 181–82.

3. U.S. Supreme Court, *In the Matter of Nancy Cruzan* (1990).

· Topic 3 ·

Autonomy of the Patient

"Burned Patient Refuses Medical Care"

$\mathcal{D}$onald "Dax" Cowart had been discharged from the U.S. Air Force after distinguished service as a fighter pilot in Vietnam. In 1973, at age twenty-five, he was severely burned in a propane gas explosion while inspecting real estate with his father. Dax and his father were rushed to the Burn Treatment Unit of Parkland Hospital in Dallas, Texas. His father died en route. Dax had severe burns over 65 percent of his body; his face and hands suffered third-degree burns, and his eyes were severely damaged. Intensive burn therapy was instituted. After an initial period during which his survival was in doubt, he stabilized. His fingers were amputated and his right eye removed. During much of his 232-day hospitalization at Parkland, his few weeks at the Texas Institute of Rehabilitation and Research at Houston, and his subsequent six-month stay at the University of Texas Medical Branch in Galveston, he repeatedly insisted that doctors cease treatment and allow him to die. Despite this demand, wound care was continued, skin grafts performed, and nutritional and fluid support provided. His mother and his family lawyer adamantly opposed his wishes. The doctors insisted first that he was unable to decide for himself, and even after a psychiatrist had declared that he was competent, they ignored his wishes, arguing that once past the pain of the acute phase and rehabilitation, Dax would realize that he could live a happy life. He was discharged from treatment totally blind, with minimal use of his hands, badly scarred, and dependent on others to assist in personal functions.

Medical and surgical treatment of severe burns rapidly improved after World War II. By 1970, patients like Dax survived burns that would certainly have killed them only a decade before. Dax, however, did not judge this sophisticated treatment of severe burns a benefit. Being kept alive was, in his view, a harm. He wanted his doctors to let him die of infection that would certainly occur once treatment was discontinued. His doctors judged that they could not ethically accede to his demand. They were obliged to sustain his life. To do otherwise would be complicity in his suicide or an act of euthanasia, long prohibited by law and medical ethics.

Dax Cowart appears in a film about his ordeal. He is severely disfigured and disabled, but his life has been a success. He went to law school and practices real estate law. He has married. Still, he eloquently defends his belief that his request to die should have been honored by his doctors. Students in bioethics courses are deeply moved by this film but vigorously debate whether Dax or his doctors (who express their views in the film) were right. One thing, however, is not open to debate: in the thirty years since his ordeal, the principle of patient autonomy has become firmly established at the heart of medical practice. The answer to the question Who decides? is now clearly the patient. The patient decides not only about life-sustaining treatment but also about every treatment that physicians propose. The principle, however, is often difficult to sustain in practice.

Dax's story, appearing at the very beginning of bioethics, reveals one of bioethics' central features: the demise of medical paternalism and the rise of patient autonomy. Paternalism means literally acting with the authority of a father, or as the *Oxford Dictionary* defines it, "limiting the freedom of the subject by well-meaning regulations." Paternalism was standard practice in traditional medical ethics. The Hippocratic physician was admonished, "Perform all your duties calmly and adroitly, concealing most things from the patient. . . . Give necessary orders with cheerfulness and serenity, turning his attention away from what is being done . . . sometimes reprove sharply and emphatically, sometimes comfort with solicitude and attention, revealing nothing of the patient's future or present condition."[1] Nothing in traditional medical ethics required the physician to respect the patient's preferences about treatment. Although British and American law did require doctors to get permission to touch or invade the patient's body, the law imposed no duty to explain the reason. Doctors clearly knew best, and it was best to follow the doctor's orders.

The switch from traditional medical ethics, based on paternalism, to bioethics, with its central tenant of patient autonomy, was a radical break with the past. The earliest bioethicists strongly supported the right of patients to choose. Theologian Joseph Fletcher stated as the thesis of his pioneering *Morals and Medicine* (1954), written two decades before Dax's ordeal, "Choice and responsibility are the very heart of ethics and the sine qua non of a man's moral status. . . . The dimensions of our moral responsibility expand, of necessity, with the advances made in medical science and medical technology. . . . [So,] in any discussion of morals and medicine, it becomes necessary to trace our moral freedom, our human action, in a number of decisions over life and death." He carried this thesis through the problems of the patient's right to know the truth about his or her condition (a right rarely recognized at that time), the right to use contraceptives (at that time illegal in many states), to conceive a child by artificial insemination (widely condemned by churches as immoral) and "to receive a merciful death from a medically competent euthanasiast" (then almost universally viewed as murder).[2]

While the centrality of "choice and responsibility as the very heart of ethics" had been a growing concept in moral philosophy since the Enlightenment, British philosopher John Stuart Mill had asserted it very boldly. He opened his groundbreaking essay *On Liberty* (1859) with the words, "one very simple principle [is] entitled to govern absolutely the dealings of society with the individual in the way of compulsion and control. . . . That principle is that the sole end for which mankind are warranted, individually or collectively, in interfering with the liberty of action in any of their number is self-protection."[3] Mill argued that others have no right to limit the freedom of a person, even if that limitation is for the good of the person. One might warn a walker that he is about to step onto a fragile bridge but may not detain him physically if he willingly chooses to proceed (if the walker has a child by the hand, he may be restrained, since the child is not willingly putting himself in danger). Mill's principle repudiates paternalism, allowing it only when harm comes to others through one's free actions.

Mill's principle is not, as he claimed, "a simple" one. It is very complex in concept and in application. Philosophers and legal scholars argue endlessly about it. Still, it is consistent with a profound strain in Anglo-American culture. For the English, every man's home has long been his castle; for the Americans, the liberty to pursue happiness is embedded in spirit, custom, and law. It is an obvious implication of the dignity of the individual that is valued so highly in both cultures. The two leading American moral philosophers, William James and John Dewey, placed human intentions, purposes, plans, and choices at the heart of morality. Thus, the absence of this liberty in the world of medicine seemed egregious to many commentators. In 1980, Ian Kennedy read his prestigious Reith lectures on the BBC (later published as *The Unmasking of Medicine*) in which he castigated the British medical profession for assuming authority over the moral decisions rightly left to patients. As stories like Dax's accumulated, it seemed obvious that a new principle must be added to medical ethics. It came to be called the *principle of respect for autonomy*, defined by Tom Beauchamp and James Childress as "acknowledging decision-making rights and enabling persons to act autonomously, whereas disrespect for autonomy involves attitudes and actions that ignore, insult or demean others' rights of autonomy. . . . To respect an autonomous agent is, at a minimum, to acknowledge that person's right to hold views, to make choices, and to take actions based on personal values and beliefs."[4]

INFORMED CONSENT

The practical implication of this principle requires that persons be honestly informed of their medical condition and about the various options that exist to deal with it. In 1914, Justice Benjamin Cardozo of the New York Court of Appeals had uttered the ringing proclamation, "Every human being of adult years and sound mind has a right to determine what shall be done with his own body; and a surgeon who performs an operation without his patient's consent, commits an assault."[5] He was reasserting an ancient rule of the English common law, namely, that invasion of another's property was trespass and of another's body was assault, unless consent was given. However, the justice said nothing about information. It took another fifty years for American courts to recognize that consent was meaningless without information. In the United States and Canada, the legal standard that governed the physician's disclosure of information was what a reasonable patient would wish to know in order to decide whether to receive treatment or not. In Britain, courts still maintain an older standard: what a reasonable practitioner would consider relevant for a patient to know. However, in all these jurisdictions, consent must be accompanied by information.

Hesitantly, and somewhat clumsily, physicians became more forthcoming in discussing diagnoses and therapies. It became common to describe informed consent as a clear, honest explanation of the nature of the patient's medical condition and the options for treatment with their attendant risks and benefits, followed by a request for permission to proceed with a course chosen by the patient. Once informed consent is acknowledged in principle, a number of practical problems appear: How do we deal with persons whose capacity to decide is compromised by mental deficit? How much information should be given? How can the informing physician ascertain whether the patient comprehends? Can patients, distressed by their illness, ever truly comprehend or choose rationally? Are there exceptions to the rule of informed consent? Should cultural differences about information and truth telling affect informed consent?

One major problem about the principle of autonomy and the practice of informed consent is the sad fact that in clinical medicine, patients are often not capable of making autonomous choices. The principle confronts persons who are unconscious, who are too immature to make decisions, or who are disoriented and distressed by pain. Still, respect for autonomy is a moral principle that applies to all humans, regardless of condition. Certainly, it cannot always be applied by going through the steps of informed consent. It has become customary in medicine to rely on the deliberation and decisions of others. For centuries, those others were the doctors treating the disabled patient. They were guided by the paternalistic ethic expressed in the Hippocratic oath: "I will act for the benefit of the sick according to my ability and judgment." In the era of bioethics, that paternalism is supplemented by the judgment of parties who have, by familial relationship or legal charge, the duty to make a "surrogate" decision.

In the cases described in topics 1 and 2, the patients, Terri Schiavo and Karen Ann Quinlan, were incapacitated: neither could engage in the discourse required for informed consent. The bioethical and biolegal literature is filled with similar cases, describing varying degrees of incapacity. Often these cases are about infants and children. Both in the clinic and in the court, the question Who should decide? is taken very seriously. Often there are customary precedents—the closest relatives are the appropriate decision makers; sometimes law establishes the rules—a court-appointed guardian or a legislatively prescribed list of surrogates is provided. A relatively recent practice, the durable power of attorney for health care, has been legally sanctioned in many jurisdictions. This empowers an individual to appoint a person to make decisions for him or her in case of the individual's incapacity. That appointed person supersedes family members and becomes the patient's official spokesperson to the doctors.

Bioethics and law also set standards for surrogate decisions. Above all, a surrogate must act in accord with the expressed or implied wishes of the person, if any are known. The courts have, in some cases, required the surrogate to offer "clear and convincing evidence" of the patient's wishes. If wishes are not known, the surrogate must conscientiously form a "best-interest" judgment, that is, consider what course is best for the person, given his or her age, capabilities, disabilities, and social setting. Sometimes such a judgment is clear enough and indisputable; at other times, considerable debate is stimulated. Yet, the insistence on the patient's interest, not the family's or the doctor's or the institution's, keeps the autonomy of the patient, now lost in fact, at the center of the debate. It is the person lying in this bed for whom life or death must be beneficial.

Bioethics has encouraged the establishment of ethics committees in hospitals. These committees, made up of various health professionals and some public members, undertake to assist in the difficult debates about appropriate ethical decisions. Usually, these debates concern best-interests arguments. Moving the debate from the distressed and heated atmosphere of a dispute between doctors and families to the cool setting of an impartial committee often helps to provide perspective, different views, and comparisons with similar cases. Misunderstanding about the medical facts may be dispelled; legal points may be clarified. The committees do not make decisions; those remain with the responsible surrogates and the doctors. The committee offers counsel. Ethics committees are a useful contribution that bioethics has made to health care.

Informed consent is but a message delivered in the course of a complex human relationship. The encounter between physician and patient, sometimes transitory, sometimes sustained, carries many meanings. It involves a worried person consulting a counselor, a hurting person calling for a healer, an afflicted person engaging an expert. It requires trust, comprehension, and empathy. Informed consent provides some essential information, but it must be delivered within this larger relationship. The skills of doctors in crafting this larger relationship arise from their personalities, complemented by experience and education. The need for such education has inspired the realm of medical humanities, a close relative of bioethics.

Had Dax argued his case in 2004 instead of 1973, many of the issues would have been clearer. The right of a competent patient to refuse even life-saving care would have been defined in ethics and in the law. Morally relevant distinctions have been drawn between acts that differ in intention, in form of action, and in consequences so that it is unlikely that one of Dax's doctors would say today, as he did in 1973, that it would be murder to cease treatment. However, certain aspects of Dax's case would be as problematic today as they were then. To what extent can a seriously traumatized patient make informed decisions? How should physicians incorporate the wishes of family members, particularly those who may be the appropriate surrogates for the patient during times of incapacity? How can physicians communicate the prospects for future life to a person so radically disabled as Dax was in the early days of his treatment? How can all parties rationally reflect on so emotional a decision? Bioethics has clarified many of the conceptual questions but can at best only articulate them. The answers must be given in each situation, in accord with the best judgment of all parties involved.

Dax's case was a telling moment in early bioethics. The principle of autonomy had not worked its way into the thinking of doctors, and few legal cases had given it weight. The principle of respect for autonomy has forced a fundamental change in the relationship between physicians and patients. It supports the right of a patient to know and to decide about what physicians will do for them. It shifts authority from medical values to personal values.

Yet, this fundamental change and its acknowledgment in law may itself be somewhat problematic. Indeed, while autonomy empowers the patient, it may also undermine the trust that must cement the therapeutic relationship. It also may encourage patients to demand that their doctor provide treatments that are unlikely to help and may harm them. In addition, it is a mistake to limit the principle of autonomy to "allowing the patient to make the decision." In its deeper philosophical sense, it is a recognition of the dignity of each person, calling for each person to deal with every other person as a distinct individual, with a history and values that are uniquely his or hers. Finally, autonomy, while a central principle of ethics and bioethics, is not the sole principle. Beneficence, nonmaleficence, and justice are also relevant to ethical decisions. We shall see these principles exemplified in the remaining topics.

NOTES

1. Works of Hippocrates, "The Decorum, xiv."
2. Joseph Fletcher, *Morals and Medicine* (Princeton, NJ: Princeton University Press, 1954), 10–12, 25.
3. J. S. Mill, *On Liberty*, ed. C. Shields (New York: Bobbs-Merrill, 1954).
4. T. Beauchamp and J. Childress, *Principles of Biomedical Ethics* (New York: Oxford University Press, 2001), 63.
5. *Schloendorff v. New York Hospital*, 1914.

BIBLIOGRAPHY

Beauchamp, T. L., and J. F. Childress. 2001. *Principles of Biomedical Ethics*, ch. 3. New York: Oxford University Press.
Berg, W., P. S. Appelbaum, C. W. Lidz, and L. S. Parker. 2001. *Informed Consent. Legal Theory and Clinical Practice*. New York: Oxford University Press.
Faden, R., and T. Beauchamp. 1986. *A History and Theory of Informed Consent*. New York: Oxford University Press.
Halpern, J. 2001. *From Detached Concern to Empathy: Humanizing Medical Practice*. New York: Oxford University Press.
Katz, J. 1984. *The Silent World of Doctor and Patient*. New Haven, CT: Yale University Press.
Kennedy, I. 1991. "The Patient on the Clapham Omnibus." In *Treat Me Right: Essays in Medical Law and Ethics*, ed. I. Kennedy. Oxford: Clarendon Press.
Kennedy, I. 1981. *The Unmasking of Medicine*. London: Allen and Unwin.
McLean, S. 1989. *A Patient's Right to Know*. Aldershot, UK: Dartmouth Publishing.

O'Neill, O. 2002. *Autonomy and Trust in Bioethics.* New York: Cambridge University Press.

Reich, W., ed. 1995. "Informed Consent." *Encyclopedia of Bioethics.* New York: Macmillan.

Schneider, C. 1998. *The Practice of Autonomy: Patients, Doctors and Medical Decisions.* New York: Oxford University Press.

Euthanasia

"Paralyzed Woman Wishes to Starve to Death"

Elizabeth Bouvia has suffered the afflictions of cerebral palsy since birth. She is quadriplegic, almost completely paralyzed except for slight facial and head movements and some motion of fingers. She is confined to bed and depends on helpers for all her needs. She also suffers from painful arthritis. Elizabeth is very intelligent and articulate. Despite her disabilities, she has attained a college degree. At age twenty-eight, she checked into a public hospital for pain relief treatment. She informed her doctors that she had decided to die and did not wish to be fed. The hospital objected and obtained a court order to feed her forcibly. Elizabeth appealed the order, and finally the California Court of Appeals granted her wish. (Ms. Bouvia then chose not to avail herself of this right and still lives.)

One major implication of informed consent is informed dissent. A person, on learning that he or she has cancer and can receive surgical, radiological, or chemotherapeutic treatments, may choose one over the others or none at all. An informed dissent may be a refusal of every form of care that results in the patient's death. Dax Cowart made that choice, and it was not granted. In the case of Elizabeth Bouvia, the court quoted the words of a presidential commission on bioethics: "the voluntary choice of a competent and informed patient should determine whether or not life-sustaining therapy will be undertaken."[1] In the past, physicians commonly believed that they were morally obliged to ignore a patient's refusal of needed care. Many also believed that a patient's death due to a doctor's discontinuing life-supporting treatment constituted homicide, or at least complicity in suicide. However, once the legal and ethical right to consent

48

to care had been acknowledged, the right to refuse care and to die seemed a logical consequence.

Refusal of life-saving care seems to most people anomalous: it is not uncommon to assume that anyone who would do such a thing must be crazy. This was the usual reaction of doctors and nurses in emergency departments when a severely bleeding patient refused blood transfusion, claiming that taking blood was contrary to God's will. This strange occurrence began to happen in the 1930s, when blood transfusion was becoming a safe and effective lifesaver. The small Christian sect of Jehovah's Witnesses found biblical texts that they interpreted as forbidding a believer to accept blood. Despite their protests, they were frequently transfused on the grounds that they were incompetent to make a reasonable choice (how could choice of death be reasonable?). Slowly, judges sided with the Witnesses, viewing their objection, however unusual, as a reasonable exercise of their religious beliefs, about which they, the judges, had no authority to rule. Today, the choice of a Jehovah's Witness is respected, except when adults attempt to refuse transfusions for children.

However, refusal of lifesaving care may be motivated by other reasons. Some persons may decide that the quality of their life is so diminished that life is no longer worth living. This conclusion may be the result of unrelieved pain, as in Elizabeth's case, or because some persons consider the prospect of deterioration or the loss of spouse or friends unacceptable or judge their lives to be a burden to others. Some persons attempt suicide to solve their problem. Others who come to this conclusion are terminally ill and under the care of a physician. They may request that their physician cause their death quickly and painlessly. In other cases, patients may be incapable of expressing such a desire to anyone, yet appear to suffer so much that some other person, a friend, family member, or care provider, may feel compelled to end their apparent suffering by causing their death.

A long debate surrounds this very human situation. Ancient Roman writers often counseled those suffering from incurable and painful disease to end their lives. Christian and Jewish teachers, however, totally repudiated that counsel. To take one's own life or to allow oneself to die when death could be avoided counted as suicide. Christian and Jewish morality condemned suicide and, by implication, suicide aided by a physician. These teachers urged sufferers to await the angel of death, sent in God's own time. This almost universal teaching prevailed until the Enlightenment, when a religious scholar and poet, John Donne, wondered whether relief of suffering by the deliberate death of the sufferer might be a virtuous rather than a vicious act, and rationalist thinker David Hume ridiculed the logic of awaiting God's call: could not the decision to take one's own life constitute that call? Despite doubts such as these, public morality and medical ethics condemned suicide with a physician's aid (although, doubtless, many physicians must have quietly hastened their patients' ends).

During the late nineteenth and early twentieth century, medicine had changed radically. An improved science of pathology began to sharpen diagnostic skills. It became possible for early diagnosis to predict the inevitability of some deadly diseases, such as cancer. The patient would have to live with the knowledge of a future, painful end. In the early twentieth century, surgical removal of tumors saved persons otherwise doomed to quick death, leaving them, often enough, to die of recurrent disease. In the 1930s, insulin stopped diabetes in its course to early death but did not eliminate its ravages on the body. At the end of the 1940s, the first antibiotics repelled lethal infection. Penicillin banished pneumonia, called by Dr. William Osler "the old man's friend," for its silent relief from the throes of death. Tuberculosis, "captain of the legions of death," in Dr. Osler's words, almost disappeared from the fray. Devastating epidemic diseases, such as polio, yielded to perfected immunization. By the 1950s, physicians could prescribe drugs to control hypertension. Chemotherapy could retard the devastation of many cancers. Surgeons moved boldly into the heart and the brain. Anesthesia and respiratory support were the beneficiaries of wartime research. By the 1960s, organ transplantation had begun, and mechanical technologies like the respirator, the pacemaker, and the dialysis machine could support seriously damaged major organs. Medicine became what it had never before been: a science and an art of sustaining life.

Euthanasia partisans noted that the ability to diagnose lethal disease in the absence of effective treatment condemned many persons to a lingering death. In light of all these changes, the Voluntary Euthanasia Legislation Society was founded in the 1930s in Great Britain. In 1936, it was influential in bringing to the House of Lords a bill to legalize voluntary euthanasia. The bill was defeated after a fascinating debate in the world's oldest debating society (one of the opponents, the king's physician, was later found to have euthanized King George V). The Euthanasia Society of America was founded in 1937. It moved in a polite, persistent way to promote the passage of proeuthanasia legislation. Bills were introduced without success in many states.

The horrors of the Holocaust cast a dark cloud over even the most restrained advocacy of euthanasia. The German medical profession had expressed a broad tolerance for "mercy killing" of the incurably ill and the mentally unfit even before the Nazi ascendancy. The Nazis began systematic extermination of "useless eaters" in hospitals for the incurable and in asylums for mental patients. The unrestrained horrors of genocide followed.

Although tarnished by these patent evils, "mercy killing" was still advo-
cated by some serious and compassionate persons. Pioneer bioethicist Joseph
Fletcher, an early member of the Euthanasia Society, devoted a chapter to euthanasia in his *Morals and Medicine* (1954). He argues that the values of personhood and autonomy should prevail over mere prolongation of life. He criticizes the traditional moral condemnation of suicide and differentiates the
motives and ends of euthanasia from those of murder. He refutes the claim
that a natural death alone is the sign that God is calling the sufferer: God,
who made humans rational, would accept a rational choice to leave life. He
repudiates other common arguments against euthanasia: it should be prohibited because physicians can make mistakes about prognosis; patients can make
impulsive decisions. He makes an impassioned plea for voluntary euthanasia
in terminal illness as a rational, courageous, and compassionate deed. Philosophers and theologians began to revisit a matter that had seemed closed. In
these discussions, the scholarly opinion moved perceptibly toward a conception of voluntary euthanasia that repudiated mercy killing of unconsenting
persons but endorsed the right of competent persons in pain and nearing
death to receive aid in ending their lives. The growing primacy of the principle of autonomy supported this significant shift of opinion.

FORGOING LIFE SUPPORT (PASSIVE EUTHANASIA)

But the new medical technologies changed the argument. In an era where
medicines were marginally effective, forgoing treatment was only peripherally
associated with the patient's death: the disease simply ran its natural course.
In the new era of effective technologies, stopping a treatment that was clearly
supporting life seemed clearly to be causing death. It became important to
sort out various kinds of euthanasia. The first distinction was between *passive*
and *active euthanasia* (these terms are rather confusing and are rarely used in
bioethics today, but they remain common in ordinary discussion). Passive euthanasia described the problem facing doctors, patients, and families when
the patient's life was supported by technology. This was the problem popu-
larized by the ugly phrase "pulling the plug."

Karen Ann Quinlan had a plug to pull; more properly, the switch controlling her ventilator could be turned off, or the tube in her larynx could be
withdrawn. Elizabeth Bouvia and Terri Schiavo had no plug: neither was
attached to a mechanical ventilator. Terri's intravenous feeding tube could
be taken out; Elizabeth would simply stop taking the spoonfuls of gruel that
were her only nutrition. Many such tragic cases, widely reported in the

media, were litigated in the courts and, more commonly, lived out in the quiet desperation of homes and hospitals.

It seemed that allowing individuals to die, when treatment offered no hope of recovery and when the wishes of the patient could be reasonably interpreted, had passed from legal and moral disapprobation to acceptance. In the Quinlan case, the justices cited with approval the Catholic doctrine (the Quinlans were Catholics) that Karen Ann's death, subsequent to removal of the respirator, would constitute the morally acceptable termination of "extraordinary means," a long-standing theological doctrine reaffirmed by Pope Pius XII in 1958. An extraordinary means was, in the theologians' definition, "any medicines, treatments and operations which cannot be obtained without excessive expense, pain or inconvenience for the patient or for others, or which, if used, would not offer a reasonable hope of benefit to the patient."[2]

In 1988, the American Medical Association (AMA) approved a statement: "For humane reasons, with informed consent, a physician may do what is medically necessary to alleviate severe pain, or cease or omit treatment to permit a terminally ill patient whose death is imminent to die. However, he should not intentionally cause death." In the same year, the British Medical Association declared that allowing a patient to die was an act of medical discretion. Thus, passive euthanasia accomplished by forgoing the treatments that sustained the life of a terminally ill person, with their consent or the permission of an authorized proxy, came to be seen as an ethically and legally accepted practice. It is commonly described today not as passive euthanasia but as "foregoing life-supporting technologies."

In one area of medical care, this problem is common and excruciating. Neonatal intensive care is a highly technical set of procedures designed to rescue very small premature infants from almost certain death. Sophisticated interventions to support the immature lungs of these infants often stave off death, but it is not uncommon, especially as smaller and smaller babies are treated, that tiny patients suffer serious problems such as severe brain hemorrhages. The prospect for these babies is dismal—they will survive, but mentally damaged—but the prospect is also uncertain. For example, a baby is born in the twenty-fifth week of pregnancy, weighing 680 g (1 lb., 7 oz.), unresponsive, and with a faint heart rate. The neonatologist initiates resuscitation but stops after ten minutes because there is no response. Some minutes later, the baby, cradled in its mother's arms, begins to cry. Resuscitation is again attempted, this time successfully, but the baby's brain, long without oxygen, is terribly damaged. Should resuscitation have been started, stopped, started again? Who decides and based on what criteria? Babies cannot exercise the principle of autonomy, and parents are obliged to promote the welfare of their child. Yet, those judgments are clouded by uncertainty and agony. Is the child's welfare served by allowing it to die? By preserving life with certain or probable damage? Rarely is the way out of these agonizing ethical dilemmas clear, and never is it easy.

AID IN DYING (ACTIVE EUTHANASIA)

A quite different problem came to be called active euthanasia. Here, although the patient's life may not be supported by any technology that can be withdrawn, being alive has become more burdensome than the patient can bear. The patient requests someone, physician or relative, to cause the patient's death by a positive act, such as suffocating, shooting, giving lethal drugs, or overdosing with sedating drugs. While passive euthanasia could be seen as allowing a patient to die a natural death, unencumbered by supporting technology, active euthanasia is poised on the brink of homicide. Even a merciful motive does not justify it (although many juries have found grounds to excuse the perpetrator). In recent years, a vigorous debate has forced reconsideration of the view that assisting a terminally ill person to die is simply and unequivocally homicide.

Some philosophers and physicians have wondered how a decision to omit life-sustaining treatment is not equivalently "intentionally causing death." Some authors have questioned the logical and psychological validity of the distinction between "active" and "passive," "omission" and "commission." In a one-page essay, "It's Over, Debbie," appearing in the *Journal of the American Medical Association*, an anonymous physician-author told a story (whether true or fictional, no one knew) about helping a dying woman to die more quickly by administering a heavy dose of morphine. That brief essay stirred up a storm of dispute among physicians and was, in the view of many observers, the spur to a more open discussion of active euthanasia within the profession.[3] The Hemlock Society was formed. Its leader published a book, *Final Exit*, that not only argued for legal euthanasia but also provided directions and recipes for those who chose such an exit. A retired pathologist, Dr. Jack Kevorkian, began to solicit patients who wished him to terminate their lives; only after a hundred highly publicized deaths was "Dr. Death" successfully prosecuted and convicted of homicide. Many persons, certainly including some jurors in his several trials, sympathized with his cause.

The principal ethical arguments surrounding active euthanasia can be sifted out of the debate. Opponents argue the following:

1. Prohibition of the direct taking of human life, except in self-defense or in the defense of others, has been a central tenet of the Judeo-Christian

tradition. It has been equally strong in the secular ethic. An ancient maxim of the Western legal tradition states that even the consent of the victim is not a defense against homicide.

2. Medical ethics has traditionally emphasized the saving and preservation of life and the improvement of its quality and has repudiated the direct taking of life. The Hippocratic oath states, "I will not administer a deadly poison to anyone when asked to do so nor suggest such a course." Contemporary organized medicine reaffirms this tradition. The Council on Ethical and Judicial Affairs of the AMA states, "Active euthanasia . . . is not a part of the practice of medicine with or without the consent of the patient." The British Medical Association states that active killing, even when requested by the patient, is unethical and should remain illegal.

3. The dedication of the medical profession to the welfare of patients and to the promotion of health might be seriously undermined in the eyes of the public and of patients by physicians' complicity in the death of the very ill, even of those who request it. It is possible that subtle changes would enter into the relationship between patients and their physicians should such a practice become common.

4. Requests for death may not be reliable because they are often made in circumstances of extreme distress, which may be alleviated by skillful pain management and other positive interventions such as those employed in hospice care.

5. Even if physician-assisted suicide is limited to the voluntary situation, it is possible that once established, the practice might become more acceptable with involuntary patients who "would have requested" to die if they had been able. Similarly, the availability of quick death may subtly coerce persons who feel that their invalid state is a burden to others. Thus, even when effecting a swift death at the request of a suffering patient seems merciful and benevolent, the acceptance of the practice as ethical may bear the seeds of frightening social consequences. In the first half of the twentieth century, many benevolent physicians supported the "euthanasia" program initiated in Germany. This practice was first directed only toward the incurably ill; it gradually expanded into genocide. Ethicists call this a slippery-slope argument; in other words, tolerance for a practice on the grounds that it is harmless will lead gradually to the toleration of more harmful practices, either by accustoming people to the values involved in the practice or by the logical extension of the argument.

Proponents of assisting patients to die offer countervailing arguments:

1. Autonomous individuals have moral authority over their lives and should be allowed the means to end them, including enlisting the assistance of those who can do so painlessly and efficiently. This is the ultimate exercise of respect for the autonomy of the patient.
2. The commonly invoked distinctions between "killing" and "allowing to die" and between "acting" and "refraining" are spurious and can be dissolved by careful philosophical analysis; thus, termination of treatment and direct killing are morally the same and, if the former is permitted, the latter should be also.
3. No person should be coerced into bearing the burdens of pain and suffering, and those who relieve people of such burdens, at their request, are acting ethically, that is, out of compassion and respect for autonomy.
4. Often the burdens of pain and disability are the result of "successful" medical intervention that has extended life; doctors who have effected this result have an obligation to respect the patient's desire no longer to bear so unrewarding a result.
5. The maxim of the Hippocratic oath is outdated because earlier medicine could never have anticipated the ability to extend dying that medicine has today. The maxim should be reinterpreted, as it is in the one modern version, the World Medical Association's Declaration of Geneva: "I will maintain the utmost respect for human life."

For these reasons, some influential voices in the medical profession, which has been generally opposed to active euthanasia, have recently expressed reasoned, carefully circumscribed support. They suggest that with proper regulation, abuses can be avoided. It is better, they believe, that skilled, sympathetic physicians aid persons to die rather than that suicide be left to the distressed patient or euthanasia to clumsy relatives or friends. It is as much a doctor's duty to relieve pain as to prevent death.

The contemporary debate has abandoned the term *euthanasia* and its distinctions. It prefers *aid-in-dying* or *physician-assisted suicide*. Aid-in-dying designates a situation in which a patient requests a physician to administer a lethal drug. The agent causing death is the physician. In physician-assisted suicide, patients request a prescription and kill themselves by taking the drug. The patient is the agent of his or her own death. By far the most important implication of defining the issue in this way is the emphasis on the choice of the agent, reflecting the dominant theme of American bioethics, respect for the autonomy of persons.

Administration of a lethal drug presumably constitutes an act of homicide; however, prescribing drugs that the patient can take at will removes the physician from direct participation. The decision and the action of ending life remain in the patient's control. The patient, then, commits suicide, which is not an illegal act under American or British law, although assistance in suicide is a criminal act. Physicians who assist a dying patient in dying should be exempted from prosecution, say advocates. Physician participation, these advocates claim, is in fact a proper medical duty of the relief of pain. This physician-assisted suicide has increasingly become the preferable way of presenting the issue.

In the 1980s, the Netherlands initiated a novel experiment. Legal authorities and the medical establishment agreed that, in cases where a dying patient with intractable pain requested medical help to hasten death, cooperating physicians would not be prosecuted. After years of experience with and debate over this approach, the Dutch parliament officially sanctioned the practice. Several major studies have reported that annually about five hundred people choose physician-assisted suicide; another two thousand choose passive euthanasia. Some evidence of a slippery slope has appeared: despite the legal controls, a significant number of deaths represent persons who, although unable to make a competent request, were caused to die by morphine administration.

By the early 1990s, American proponents of active, voluntary euthanasia had generated enough popular strength to introduce initiatives in the states of Washington (1991), California (1992), and Oregon (1995) that would legally authorize physicians to hasten the deaths of requesting, competent, terminal patients. The Washington and California initiatives narrowly failed, but the citizens of Oregon accepted (also narrowly) the Death with Dignity Act, granting that "an adult may make a written request for medication for the purpose of ending his or her life in a humane and dignified manner." During the first four years after legalization (1998–2001), some seventy Oregonians sought this assistance, comprising about 0.35 percent of all deaths from similar diseases. There is little evidence that physicians or patients have abused the law.

The legal tolerance of the Dutch and Oregonians is not matched elsewhere. The U.S. Supreme Court reviewed a case brought by several terminally ill persons and their physicians who claimed that their constitutionally guaranteed liberties were impeded by state law criminalizing assisted suicide. The justices determined that no protected constitutional liberty was infringed and that individual states could outlaw assisted suicide, although several justices expressed sympathy for the suffering and even hinted that American society may someday tolerate the practice (*Washington v. Glucksberg, Vacco v. Quill,* 1997). The British parliament rejected bills to legalize active euthanasia in 1936, 1969, and 1990. In 2002, Diane Pretty, a forty-year-old woman, paralyzed by motoneuron disease (amatrophic lateral sclerosis) sought permission from British courts for her husband to end her life. The High Court, Court of Appeals, and the House of Lords denied her petition. She carried it to the European Court of Human Rights, which refused to acknowledge that British law prohibiting assisted suicide violated her right not to be subjected to "inhumane or degrading treatment" proscribed in the European Convention on Human Rights. In Spain, the dramatic 1998 suicide of Ramon Sampedro, paralyzed after a dive into shallow water, stirred support for assisted suicide in that Catholic land. Thus, although sympathy for those suffering the trials of terminal or chronic illness is widespread and ethical arguments in favor of their relief can be compelling, law throughout the world is reluctant to open that door. (Belgium and Switzerland have recently enacted law similar to the Netherlands.)

Even should assisted suicide be legalized, individual physicians will have to make conscientious decisions about whether to assist patients in ending their lives. Some physicians will refrain on grounds of conscientious objection. The practice of physician-assisted suicide will require difficult decisions about what constitutes decisional capacity and terminal illness and whether all means of relieving pain have been exhausted. In particular, limiting legal authorization to only competent patients in terminal illness will raise questions about those in equally distressing circumstances who are unable to request or self-administer lethal medication and about persons who are not terminal but who anticipate slow death from degenerative disease.

Dr. Cecily Saunders founded the first hospices in England in the 1960s. These institutions took seriously the care of the terminally ill. Specializing in palliative care, the relief of pain, they brought patients physical comfort and spiritual support. The application of intensive, life-saving interventions was avoided. The hospice movement has spread around the world and now takes many forms in many places. Palliative care is becoming recognized as a medical specialty. In arguments about euthanasia, opponents often suggest that more effective palliative care reduces the need and the desire for assisted death.

Assisted suicide should not be debated without reflecting on the social situation in which seriously ill persons receive medical care. The failure of the medical system to include all who need help, the inadequacy of palliative care for pain, the lack of personal physicians for many patients, and other features of the medical-care system can color the manner in which persons perceive the end of life. Social institutions, such as hospice, that can alleviate the burdens of dying must be supported. The structures of social institutions that surround death and dying must be such that both compassion can be found and personal autonomy expressed. Today, Dax might have had his treatment stopped at his request. He would then have faced a lingering death, possibly in great pain.

Today, Elizabeth Bouvia's feeding might cease, but she would starve to death. Both could, conceivably, ask for a quick ending, aided by a skillful physician. Their request would not be heard (at least publicly or unless both lived in Oregon or Holland). The debate over assisted suicide goes on.

NOTES

1. *Bouvia v. Superior Court*, California Court of Appeals, 1986; President's Commission for the Study of Ethical Problems in Medicine, "Deciding to Forego Life-Sustaining Treatment" (1983), in *Source Book in Bioethics*, ed. A. Jonsen, R. Veatch, and L. Walters (Washington, DC: Georgetown University Press), 160.

2. G. Kelly, *Medico-Moral Problems* (St. Louis, MO: Catholic Hospital Association, 1958), 135; Pope Pius XII, "Discourse to Anesthesiologists," *The Pope Speaks*, 1958, 393–98.

3. "It's Over, Debbie," *Journal of the American Medical Association* 259 (1988): 272.

BIBLIOGRAPHY

Beauchamp, T. 1996. *Intending Death*. Upper Saddle River, NJ: Prentice Hall.

Beauchamp, T., and J. Childress. 2001. *Principles of Biomedical Ethics*, ch. 4. New York: Oxford University Press.

Foley, K., and H. Hendin, eds. 2002. *The Case against Assisted Suicide*. Baltimore: Johns Hopkins University Press.

Glover, J. 1977. *Causing Death and Saving Lives*. New York: Penguin Books.

Hillyard, D., and J. Dombrink. 2001. *Dying Right*. New York: Routledge, 2001.

Jonsen, A. *The Birth of Bioethics*, ch. 8. New York: Oxford University Press.

Keown, J. 2002. *Euthanasia, Ethics and Public Policy: An Argument against Legalization*. Cambridge, UK: Cambridge University Press.

Lantos, J. 2001. *The Lazarus Case: Life and Death Issues in Neonatal Intensive Care*. Baltimore: Johns Hopkins University Press.

Meisel, A. 1995. *The Right to Die*. New York: Wiley and Sons.

Quill, T., and M. Battin, eds. 2004. *Physician-Assisted Dying: The Case for Palliative Care and Patient Choice*. Baltimore: Johns Hopkins University Press.

Rachels, J. 1986. *The End of Life: Euthanasia and Morality*. New York: Oxford University Press.

Reich, W. 1995. "Death and Dying: Euthanasia and Sustaining Life," *Encyclopedia of Bioethics*. New York: Macmillan.

Steinbock, B., and A. Norcross. 1994. *Killing and Letting Die*. New York: Fordham University Press.

· Topic 5 ·

Organ Transplantation

"Miracle Transplant Kills Girl"

On February 7, 2003, a heart and two lungs, taken from a cadaver in Boston, were transplanted into seventeen-year-old Jésica Santillán at Duke University Hospital in Durham, North Carolina. A news article said, "Until that moment, Jésica had been on the brink of a miracle."[1] But, as soon as the block of organs was in place, a call from the laboratory alerted the surgeons that the blood type of the donated organs (type A) did not match Jésica's blood type (type O). Already Jésica's antibodies were attacking the transplanted heart and lungs, and an irreversible destruction had begun. A second transplant, done within hours, was too late. Jésica suffered massive bleeding into her brain. With her parent's permission, she was removed from the ventilator and died on Saturday, February 8. Who was responsible for this tragic mistake: did the surgeon who had requested the organs fail to ask about the blood type? Did the donor service supplying the organs fail to inform the transplant team? Regardless of responsibility, Jésica, smuggled from Mexico by her impoverished parents and sponsored for the transplant by a wealthy Texan contractor, had lost her last chance at life. Organ transplantation, truly a miracle of beneficence in modern medicine, can cause great harm. In Jésica's case, it was, as the news article concluded, "a miracle that fell just short."

This tragic event took place almost fifty years after organ transplantation entered the medical world. Kidneys were first transplanted in 1954, hearts in 1968, and then transplantation of many other organs followed. Transplantation was an ethical revolution: for the first time, surgeons operated on one person, the organ donor, not for his or her benefit but for the benefit of another, the recipient. For the first time, therapy depended on obtaining a vital

59

organ from one person to give to another. That very organ, with its potential for life, could also kill: its tissue, foreign to the new body, could stimulate massive and lethal immune reaction. The ancient maxim, "be of benefit and do no harm," became a conundrum: the surgeon now had two patients, one who didn't benefit from the surgery and the other whose benefit came from the harm done to the other! As is often the case, the conundrum was turned over to the philosophers. For example, the story about Jésica's death continues: "And finally, the philosophers will get to weigh in on the question of how to allocate the ultimate scarce resource, living human tissue. Having botched one operation, did the doctors owe Jésica a second chance at life? Or should someone have pointed out what, in retrospect, seems obvious: her chance of surviving a second operation was almost nil?"[2] Should the second set of organs go to another waiting patient whose chance of survival is much greater? Also, Jésica was an illegal immigrant: does she have any claim on an American organ? The world of organ transplantation, miraculous as it is, is filled with moral conundrums.

The pioneers of transplantation quickly recognized the moral dimensions of their enterprise. In 1964, the editor of the *Annals of Internal Medicine* wrote a provocative article pointing out the "social and moral problems inherent in . . . advances that hold great hope for many patients with organs diseased beyond any chance of healing and repair." Among those problems were the failure of the procedures to live up to expectations, the necessity of choosing among patients, and the great social investment required to "prolong for an uncertain period the lives of a relatively few people." Letters from the leaders of transplant medicine flooded the journal. All correspondents agreed with the editor's concerns. Most of them confessed they had, in the words of Dr. Joseph Murray, the first successful transplanter of kidneys, given "a great deal of soul searching to these problems." One writer suggested "a study of these problems by scholarly specialists of high renown from the fields of philosophy, religion, biology and the social sciences. Few physicians are sufficiently grounded in these disciplines to bring to bear the wisdom of the ages on such questions."[3]

Transplantation challenged the traditional ethic of medical paternalism, the authority of the physician as sole determiner of the course of treatment. Clearly, the donor of a kidney, or a heart, or a lung must be a fully informed participant; the recipient who will live with another's organ must also accept and appreciate this portentous fact. Yet, the precise roles of the patients and the physician in making decisions were still vague. In the early days of transplantation, one surgeon stated that "it is not enough to tell the patient that 'there is no other hope.' . . . He should be given a clear picture of the hazards involved and allowed to join in the discussion. . . . Yet under no circumstances should the final decision be left in the hands of the patient; he has not the education, the background nor dispassionate view necessary to make the decision in his own best self-interest."[4] Such a statement asserts a paternalism that would soon come under severe attack. Now, more than ever before, patients choose not simply to have an operation but to live with the consequences of that operation throughout their remaining lives.

Also, traditional medical ethics ordered doctors to do no harm unless the harm—bleeding, cauterizing, amputating—was intended to cure the patient. Since transplanters removed healthy kidneys from healthy persons, they presumably violated that ancient prohibition. Was it right to remove a healthy organ from a healthy person, even to save the life of another person? Dr. Murray himself noted that "as physicians motivated and educated to make sick people well, we make a basic qualitative shift in our aims when we risk the health of a well person, no matter how pure our motives." He hoped that the time would soon come when "even identical twins will not require a living donor."[5] (His own successes initially depended on transplanting organs between identical twins who, because they share an identical immune response, will not reject the organ.)

Many religious traditions view any foray into bodily integrity for purposes other than maintenance of personal health as morally prohibited "mutilation." In some faiths, this prohibition applies even to the bodies of the dead. Jewish religious law forbids the mutilation of the human body, even autopsy. Catholic moralists prohibit any mutilation of a healthy body. Traditionally, a necessary surgical amputation could be justified by the *principle of totality*: only the health of the total body justifies the removal of a diseased part. Thus, mutilation was justified if a person could save his life only by cutting off his hand (trapped, for example, under a fallen beam). The principle of totality was designed for amputation, the most common surgical operation of antiquity; organ transplantation was inconceivable to those antique moralists. When transplantation became feasible, some Catholic theologians recalled that Catholic doctrine, as far back as Thomas Aquinas, had seen the sacrifice of one's life for the good of another as an act of charity. Much more so, they said, was the undertaking of a risk for a proportionate benefit to another. Scholars in Rabbinic law accepted that the removal of an organ for immediate and genuine benefit of another person should not be considered a reprehensible mutilation. Indeed, Jewish law gives highest priority to the saving of life.

Pioneer bioethicist and Methodist theologian Paul Ramsey proposed a carefully circumscribed *principle of reasonable self-sacrifice*. He insists that the advantage to the recipient must be greater than the disadvantage to the donor. A strong respect for the bodily integrity and health of the donor is the only protection against the false belief that an organ belongs as much to the one as to the other. We should not consider transplantation as moving "interchangeable parts between interchangeable personal embodiments."[6] These moralists reconceptualized transplantation from an act of mutilation to an act of donation. This new concept supported the widespread public view that the giving of an organ for another's life and health was a noble and generous act; it was a "gift of life." It also reflected the principle of autonomy—with a difference: the free agent was not only making a free choice but also fulfilling the moral obligation of charity, service to others, and saving of life.

Outside the Western traditions, similar views emerged. Islamic beliefs about resurrection require bodily integrity at the time of death. Buddhism also abhors mutilation of the body, and transplantation has been viewed skeptically. Still, these religious traditions have responded to the novel situation of transplantation. In most Islamic and Buddhist countries, donation after death has been permitted if the explicit consent of the donor is obtained before death. In Japan, however, a persistent public reluctance has inhibited heart, liver, and lung transplantation, due to hesitation over criteria for defining death.

The law evolved to meet medical, ethical, and popular acceptance of transplantation. Common law had long adhered to the rigid rule that one cannot consent to be maimed. This rule failed to appreciate the unique situation of transplantation, in which the "maiming" provides a source of life for another. Increasingly, jurisprudential opinion shifted from that rigid rule to the position that if both donor and recipient are competent adults who intelligently consent to the transplantation after full explanation, there should be no legal impediment. In addition to consent, a medical judgment of relative risks to donor and recipient, a high degree of caution and concern for the donor, and the absence of alternatives to save the life of the recipient move transplantation from a suspicious trespass on the body to a common surgical procedure, permitted by both parties. Judicial rulings supported this position: many legal cases in Britain and America authorized voluntary donation.

By 1970, all American states had enacted the Uniform Anatomical Gift Act, which authorized competent adults to donate their bodily organs after their deaths by signing a legally valid document (in practice, unfortunately, this donation may be denied by relatives, a denial that is usually accepted by doctors). In the absence of such a document, specified family members could authorize donation unless the deceased has specifically denied the intent to donate. Many states allow persons to signify their willingness to donate organs by a notice on their driver's license. Although the Uniform Anatomical Gift Act applies only to organs harvested after death, it reinforces the concept that living persons had a legal right to make such a gift prior to death. In some countries, such as France, the concept of "presumed permission" prevails; that is, organs can be harvested from cadavers without advance, actual permission, unless the deceased explicitly refused to donate prior to death.

The moral theme of the era of transplantation became donation. Both the living and the dead could freely give the gift of life to another desperately ill person. Kin would strengthen the bond of love; strangers would be united by a bond of flesh. Although some worried about unwonted psychological and emotional repercussions, the "gift relationship" entered medical ethics as a new moral value. It sanctioned a formerly forbidden mutilation and provided a noble motive for offering one's organs in life or after death. The combined reflections of physicians, lawyers, and theologians had converged around a central concept that carried both moral weight and public appeal. One theologian wrote, "It is surely the mark of the most profound reverence toward one's neighbor to be willing to sacrifice—for serious reasons—an organ of one's own body for him in his necessity."[7] In the course of this technical and ethical evolution, the benefit of traditional medical ethics was stretched to reach to persons other than the patient seeking help from the doctor.

As transplantation techniques advance, transplantation of multiple organs, as in Jésica's case, becomes possible. Also, transplantation of partial livers, which can regrow in the donor and the recipient, is now done. Bone marrow and stem cells are transplanted for successful treatment of blood cancers and similar conditions. Mechanical hearts have been repeatedly implanted but without great success; research on other artificial organs is intense.

DISTRIBUTION OF ORGANS

Donation provides a moral justification for only one aspect of transplantation: it authorizes sharing gifts of life. It does not resolve how to distribute these precious and rare gifts among the many persons who need them. As the story of Jésica shows, the right organs must go to the right patients. Living and dead donors provide many fewer organs than desperate patients require. In 2002, 79,387 patients were on waiting lists for all transplantable organs; 24,544 patients received transplants; more than 6,000 patients were reported to have died while waiting. On the day this page was written, December 18, 2004, 87,345 Americans were on waiting lists for all organs: the number of expectant recipients grows, while the number of donated organs remains level. The problem of distributing organs poses the ethical question of fairness. What constitutes a just distribution of organs? How can discrimination by economic status, race, and gender be avoided? Can a system that assures fair distribution be devised? A few commentators have suggested a national harvesting of organs; a few others favor a free market in organs. Indeed, such a market came into being in India, where poor people have sold kidneys both locally and globally. Although many nations (as does the United States) forbid sale of organs, widespread organ-trafficking rings are said to exist. Most ethical writers have disdained these approaches, saying that they violate the crucial ethical principle of equity, favoring the wealthy and well placed and exploiting the poor, whose receipt of payment lifts them only briefly out of poverty and often leaves them with health problems.

The United States has devised a national system, the United Network for Organ Sharing (UNOS), designed to distribute organs nationally in accord with criteria of need and medical suitability. All persons in need of organs are registered, and notification of available organs is prompt. Systems of retrieval swiftly move kidneys and hearts from a dead person in New England to a waiting patient in the Midwest or, as in Jésica's case, from Boston to Durham. This complex computerized system reduces, even if it does not eliminate, the unjust effects of favoritism, social status, race, and gender. Also, increased efforts to encourage donation and to seek organs from the families of deceased persons are implemented: tax deductions have been offered by a few states; payment of burial costs has been suggested. Yet, even with a strong national system, equity is challenged. It seems clear that race has an effect on access to transplants. In the United States, many studies report that persons of color wait longer and are less likely to receive organs than whites. Proximity to major transplant centers and ability to navigate the complex system of transplant services also improve chances for transplantation.

Alternatives to human organs are being sought. A few surgeons have attempted to graft animal organs into human patients (xenotransplantation). This was unsuccessful. Immune reaction was devastating. Animal advocates objected, particularly to the use of baboons, an endangered species. Pig hearts are sized right for humans but harbor a virus deadly to humans. Many researchers are attempting to genetically engineer animal tissue for human use. Mechanical substitutes for hearts, which are simple pumps, have been tried, again with little success: patients may live for a month or two but then are defeated, usually by infection.

Donation provides a moral warrant to take organs from one person and give them to another. But donation also flows from moral altruism, usually found between relatives. In the early days of transplantation, genetically related relatives were indispensable donors; later, even after improved immunosuppressive medication made transplantation possible between unrelated persons, relatives continued to be the primary donors of organs. In recent years, a practice known as *nondirected donation* has appeared: persons urged solely by altruism offer a kidney, bone marrow or stem cells, or partial livers to any needy patient. They are willing to take the risks of an operation and, in the case of kidney, of living with a single kidney (usually harmless) in order to provide the gift of life to a stranger.

The idea of strangers offering kidneys or partial livers troubles some. They suspect that an altruism so extreme, in the absence of the deep emotional bonds of kinship, may be tinged by psychopathology. They also worry that attempts to encourage donation by strangers may make transplantation medicine appear predatory. Because partial-liver donors run a significant risk of death, unrelated donors are usually rejected, but kidney donors, for whom surgery is now relatively simple, have been accepted. It is difficult to condemn so obvious an example of the prime ethical principle of transplantation, donation. Indeed, some bioethicists who espouse a strict utilitarian principle, namely that the moral value of an act is assessed by that act's contribution to the greater happiness of the greater number, view nondirected donation as obligatory.

Hearts, unlike kidneys or partial livers, cannot be removed from the body without causing death. Ideally, any organ destined for transplantation should be taken from a body still vital in the organic sense: blood should be flowing and oxygen perfusing the tissues. If this is happening, however, is the donor dead, or does the excision of the heart kill the donor? An ethical and legal decision was made to define death as whole-brain death as we saw in topic 1. Thus, only persons whose brains have irreversibly ceased to function and whose circulation is artificially sustained are candidates for organ salvage. This is a small population.

Should we expand our reach for organs beyond those who meet the criteria for whole-brain death to persons in persistent vegetative state or to terminally ill persons? Some transplant institutions have inaugurated a policy of *non-heart-beating donors*, whereby terminally ill persons sustained by ventilators are sedated, taken to an operating room, and removed from the ventilator. When breathing and heart beat stop, death is declared, and the surgeon removes the organs for transplantation. Even though this policy requires the prior consent to donate, either by the person or by an appropriate proxy, some have objected that it is the first step on the slippery slope toward the "relentless expanding of the realm of sheer thinghood and unrestricted utility" that philosopher Hans Jonas saw as a consequence of the redefinition of death.[8]

The story of Jésica Santillán reveals how this complex system of distribution, built to assure justice and fairness, can go wrong. It can fail in other ways, as when the media reports that a famous person appears to jump the queue to get an organ before less famous folk. It provides little guidance when facing agonizing questions, such as giving the next available heart to a person sentenced to life imprisonment or to a patient in desperate straits due to an apparent suicide attempt (Tylenol overdoses, for example, can cause fulminant liver failure). Rather than abandon the ethical principles of donation and equity that should govern the ethics of transplantation, the systems struggle to perfect their processes. Organ transplantation is certainly one of the miracles of the new medicine—a miracle both in its technical virtuosity and in its altruism—but it needs constant tending.

NOTES

1. J. Adler, "A Tragic Error," *Newsweek* (March 3, 2003): 25.
2. Adler, "A Tragic Error," 25.
3. R. Elkington, "Moral Problems in the Use of Borrowed Organs," *Annals of Internal Medicine* 60 (1964): 309, 355.
4. Francis Moore, M.D., quoted in *The Birth of Bioethics*, ed. A. Jonsen (New York: Oxford University Press, 1998), 203.
5. In *The Law and Ethics of Transplantation*, ed. G. Woltenholme and M. O'Conner (London: J. and A. Churchill, 1966), 59.
6. P. Ramsey, *The Patient as Person: Explorations in Medical Ethics*, 2nd ed. New Haven, CT: Yale University Press, 2002), 197.
7. B. Häring, *The Law of Christ* (Westminster, MD.: Newman Press, 1964), III:242.
8. See topic 1, page 31.

BIBLIOGRAPHY

Caplan, A. 1998. *Ethics of Organ Transplantation*. New York: Prometheus.
Fox, R., and J. Swazey. 1992. *Spare Parts: Organ Replacement in American Society*. New York: Oxford University Press.
Jonsen, A. 1998. *The Birth of Bioethics*, ch. 7. New York: Oxford University Press.
Nuffield Council on Bioethics. *Animal to Human Transplants: The Ethics of Xenotransplantation*, available at www.nuffieldbioethics.org.
Reich, W., ed. 1995. "Organ and Tissue Procurement," "Organ and Tissue Transplantation," and "Xenografts," *Encyclopedia of Bioethics*. New York: Macmillan.
Veatch, R. 2002. *Transplantation Ethics*. Washington, DC: Georgetown University Press.
Youngner, S., R. Fox, and L. O'Connell. 1996. *Organ Transplantation: Meanings and Realities*. Madison: University of Wisconsin Press.

• *Topic 6* •

Assisted Reproduction

"Fertility Panic: Should You Freeze Your Eggs?"

A cover story of a fashionable magazine told the story of three women in their thirties, single and successful in business, who wanted babies—but not now. They wished to time that event to suit their careers and their feelings. All were investigating an experimental procedure, egg freezing, that "promises to prolong a woman's chance of having a baby when she is good and ready." (Frozen embryos are routinely used, but frozen ova seem vulnerable to thawing, although a few clinics have reported a few live births from frozen ova.) Several clinics offer this, as yet unproven, technique at a steep price—about $10,000. The frozen eggs, taken when the ova are still viable, can wait until the woman is "good and ready" and can select a sperm donor to create an embryo. The glitzy article was exuberant, but on the last page, a spoilsport bioethicist is introduced "to raise provocative questions." He ruminates, "if social pressure leads to everyone doing this, is that really the best use of our resources? When is it irresponsible not to freeze eggs—is it the obligation of a parent whose young daughter is undergoing surgery? . . . Then there's the most obvious [question] of all: will the babies be healthy?"[1]

The world of assisted reproductive technology (ART) depicted in the article is far different than it was on July 25, 1978, the day Leslie Brown delivered a girl baby, who was named Louise Joy. After nine years of trying to become pregnant, Mrs. Brown learned she could not conceive because her fallopian tubes had been damaged by an earlier ectopic pregnancy. Mr. and Mrs. Brown visited gynecologist Patrick Steptoe, who had been collaborating on fertility research with Cambridge physiologist, Prof. R. G. Edwards. In

their experiments, they removed ova from female animals, fertilized the re-
trieved ova under laboratory conditions (in vitro), and implanted the fertilized
embryo in the animal's womb. These scientists welcomed Mrs. Brown as their
first human research subject. Ova were taken from Mrs. Brown, fertilized
with Mr. Brown's sperm in a laboratory dish, and implanted as an embryo in
Mrs. Brown. Baby Louise, born nine months later, was christened by the media as the "first test-tube baby." The era of ART had begun.

A long-sought dream had come true, a technical remedy for infertility.
That technical remedy could bring the joy of a child to couples whose infertility was due to physical strictures of the fallopian tubes. However, that remedy stirred an ethical maelstrom. The ethics of reproduction, built around features of human life that seemed fixed and natural, encountered a strange and
seemingly unnatural novelty: the conception of a child without coitus. This
shocked the mores of the day. Also, the technique put the human conceptus
into the hands of scientists, making it possible to manipulate, design, and
"clone" human beings.

ART has become a widespread practice, with many forms. Some forty
thousand babies, or one in one hundred, born in the United States are conceived annually in this manner. ART can provide children for couples like the
Browns or for same-sex partners, for unmarried women, and for post-
menopausal women. It can retrieve gametes from a couple, married or not,
and provide a surrogate to carry the child. It can help couples select children
of a desired gender and, soon, with chosen genetic traits. It preserves and
banks frozen embryos and, as our magazine story shows, will soon stock
frozen oocytes. It can save an embryo made before chemotherapy (and perhaps even preserve prechemotherapy ovarian tissue) so that women who
might loose their fertility as they fight cancer can later have a baby. ART clinical procedures are expensive (rarely costing less than $50,000 and often up to
$300,000) and often unsuccessful (about 70 percent of single attempts fail; al-
though statistics are difficult to analyze, about 32 percent of all efforts result
in pregnancies). They are often not covered by insurance (some 85 percent of
health-insurance policies exclude ART). In the United States, ART is a
highly profitable medical industry (patients pay clinics over $1 billion a year).
The American industry is almost without legal surveillance. It is, essentially,
an unregulated medical marketplace. In the United Kingdom, the Human
Fertilisation and Embryology Authority (HFEA) was established in 1990 to
provide oversight and guidance and to license and monitor clinics and research laboratories.

Infertility, the inability to generate children, is an ancient curse. Reme-
dies for infertility abound in folk and ancient medicine. As science explored
the physiology of human reproduction in the nineteenth century, attempts to

remedy infertility became more focused and effective. Artificial insemination, injecting sperm into the vagina, was the earliest and, until Baby Louise, the only technique. In the 1880s, Dr. William Panacost in Philadelphia used donor sperm from "the handsomest medical student in the class" to impregnate a woman whose husband was infertile. This event was surrounded by the greatest secrecy and was only reported in 1909. Once revealed, it aroused more admiration than criticism (although it was assailed by clergy as "medical adultery").

Artificial insemination improved in efficacy and, as might be expected, ingenuity. Husbands, if not infertile, could donate, but commonly, other, usually anonymous men were glad to donate. Sperm was first frozen and stored in 1953, and the 1970s saw a fourfold increase in demand for donor insemination. The legal status of children born of artificial insemination was uncertain. In the United Kingdom, a committee of the Department of Health recommended as late as 1960 that the status of illegitimacy be retained for such children. A New York appellate court ruled similarly in 1963, but in 1968, the California Supreme Court granted legitimacy to a child conceived by AID, the clever acronym for artificial insemination by donor.

The Catholic Church took a firm stance against any procedure that was seen to violate the sexual process leading to conception. The Vatican in 1897 had condemned "artificial fecondation," and in 1949, Pope Pius XII made it clear that the prohibition included spousal as well as donor insemination. Even as the practice became more common medically, many religious groups remained hesitant, particularly about donor insemination. In 1973, Rev. G. R. Dunstan, professor of moral and social theology at King's College, London, noted the general skepticism of religious groups. "No Christian Church in the United Kingdom," he said, "has explicitly favored the practice and the judgment of Jewish Orthodoxy is hostile." (The rabbinate has in recent years become more approving, and ART is commonly available in Israel.) However, Dunstan deplored the deception and secrecy fostered by the legal status of illegitimacy and payment for semen.[2]

THE ETHICAL ARGUMENTS

Within a few years of Baby Louise's birth, a vast nursery of babies had come into being, some by the same process as Baby Louise, others by more elaborate manipulations. Reproductive endocrinology was surging ahead, and the dreams (and nightmares) of the past were becoming real. Questions about ownership of fertilized embryos, rightful claims of parenthood among the multiple contributors to a child's being, and preimplantation research and diagnosis were raised not in theory but in real cases. Some feminists rejoiced that reproduction had been freed from male hegemony; others deplored the exploitation of women as egg donors and surrogates. These and many other questions provided ample material for the reflections of bioethicists and for puzzled judges called upon to settle unprecedented legal problems.

Joseph Fletcher was the first bioethicist to speak. Four years before Baby Louise made the possible actual, Fletcher's book *Ethics of Genetic Control* (1974) praised the techniques of assisted reproduction for allowing rational humans to "end reproductive roulette." He considered (with remarkable prescience) the panoply of actual and possible reproductive techniques, such as artificial insemination, test-tube conceptions, artificial gestation, preselection of sex, cloning, and storage banks of embryos, and pronounced them all good. He so judged because they amplified human choice and promoted human well-being. While he glimpsed possible abuses, he judged that in general, people would properly use these enhancements of choice and welfare.[3] This opinion was typical of Dr. Fletcher's biomedical ethics but not of many others who watched the same developments.

Ethicist, biochemist, and physician Leon Kass took a diametrically opposite position. Kass asked whether we have the wisdom to manufacture babies and to deal with the broad implications that will flow from "divorcing the generation of human life from human sexuality and ultimately from the confines of the human body?" He reviewed those implications: problems raised by the disposal of spare embryos, by surrogate gestational mothers, by the commodification (commercial use) of gametes and embryos, by the desire to design "perfect" children and the depreciation of defective ones, by ambiguity over personal identity, and finally, by the dehumanization of sexuality, marriage, and procreation. He answered his question about the wisdom of making babies in these new ways with a resounding no. In his view, each problem raises so many questions to which we have not the inkling of an answer that "when we lack the sufficient wisdom . . . wisdom consists in not doing. Restraint, caution, abstention and delay are what this second best (and maybe only) wisdom dictates with respect to baby manufacture." If this wisdom not to do remained unheeded, then we must establish procedures to monitor and regulate procedures and establish "effective international control so that one nation's folly does not lead the world into degradation."[4]

Despite such portentous doubts, the science of reproductive endocrinology and its concomitant technologies rushed ahead. In vitro fertilization (IVF) quickly became a relatively simple clinical procedure, although efficiently produced pregnancies remained elusive. In short order, oocytes were not only fertilized with ease, but the resultant embryos could be frozen and stored for later implantation or for other uses. These rapid developments stimulated rapid response from the public and from policy makers.

Australia, home of a thriving reproductive science, was the first to prepare policy. In 1982, the state of Victoria established the Committee to Consider the Social, Ethical, and Legal Issues Arising from IVF. The committee agreed that "respect" was owed the human embryo but, like almost every other group that has faced these issues, provided neither a clear definition of respect nor much guidance about what it entails in practice. The report suggested that couples be given three options about disposition of embryos: donation to another couple, research use, or destruction. If destruction were chosen, removing the ampoule from the freezer to thaw would be the moral equivalent of withdrawing life support for the embryo. Research was permitted on embryos prior to fourteen days of development. The Victoria Legislature accepted the report as the basis for the Infertility Act of 1984, the world's first legislation on IVF. When faced with the question of actually destroying real embryos, the same parliament backtracked. An American couple had gone to the Melbourne Fertility Clinic and, after several failed attempts to initiate a pregnancy, had left two frozen embryos in storage for another try. Two years later, they were killed in a plane crash. Despite its earlier endorsement of the destruction of orphan embryos, Parliament, in the face of a public outcry, required that these embryos be donated to another couple.

One of England's leading moral philosophers, Mary Warnock, was appointed chair of a royal commission "to examine the social, ethical and legal implications of recent, and potential developments in the field of human assisted reproduction." After wide consultation with scientific, professional, and religious bodies and individuals, the Warnock Report appeared in June 1984. It recommended that commercial surrogacy (paying a woman to carry a baby for another woman) be made illegal. It permitted research on spare and deliberately created embryos up to the fourteenth day of development. Although lucidly written, the report made little effort to formulate justifying arguments. The underlying rationale of "respect for the fetus" was qualified as "not absolute and may be balanced against the benefits arising from research." The Warnock Report stands as an important bioethical milestone, particularly in its endorsement of a fourteen-day limit on research and manipulation of in vitro embryos. The government responded by establishing HEFA.

In the United States, the Ethics Advisory Board (EAB) of the Department of Health, Education, and Welfare was asked to consider whether the federal government should finance research on IVF. It agreed with the Warnock Report that the respect due to the human embryo is not absolute and allowed, as did Warnock, research on embryos during the first two weeks of life. The Reagan administration ignored the EAB report; no regulations or oversight emerged. As a result, the door was opened, unintentionally, to an open market in this ethically sensitive technology, in contrast to the sensible British establishment of HEFA.

IVF and embryo transfer was invented for infertile couples like the Browns. All of the policy statements recommended that IVF should be confined to married couples, a recommendation that has been widely ignored. The technology made possible many other procreative arrangements. The most obvious of these was that a woman other than the woman whose egg had been fertilized might carry the growing fetus. This practice, for which the term *surrogate mother* was coined, had already been employed for the less technical process of artificial insemination. Surrogate mothering raises ethical problems. Surrogate mothers might be loath to give up the baby they have borne; they might even claim the baby as their own. The child might be harmed by uncertainty about the identity of its parents. Monetary exchange for a baby, generally forbidden by adoption laws, raises the question of "child selling" and the danger of perceiving a child as an article of commerce (the phrase "commodification of children" was coined to express this problem).

The quiet practice of surrogate gestation became noisy with the case of Baby M. In 1985, William and Elizabeth Stern agreed to pay Mary Beth Whitehead $10,000 to bear a baby conceived by artificial insemination from Mr. Stern. After the baby, named in legalese "Baby M," was delivered, Ms. Whitehead refused to surrender the child, claiming that she was its natural mother. The Sterns sued to enforce the contract; the Supreme Court of New Jersey granted their petition. The case was followed avidly in the media, and phrases like "surrogate mother," "gestational mother," and "birth mother" entered the public vocabulary.

The Baby M case pushed all forms of surrogate motherhood—the old form by insemination and the new form by IVF and embryo transfer—into public attention. The new technology of assisted reproduction befuddled the identity of parenthood and the heritage of children even more than had artificial insemination: five or six persons could now contribute to making a baby and had some claim on the newborn child. A number of surrogacy cases came to the courts, which rendered conflicting opinions. In 2003, a British high court rejected the plea of two women who wished to use frozen embryos, created with sperm from their partners, to initiate a pregnancy. In both cases, the couples had subsequently separated, and the women's former partners refused permission to use the embryos to which they had contributed. The judge ruled that without the consent of both partners to storage and use of the embryos, they must be destroyed. In contemporary ART, best practice dictates that the couple and the clinic sign a contract in which the ownership of the embryos is designated and the disposal of spare embryos is decided; a choice between donation to another couple, use for research, or destruction is usually offered. It is estimated that about four hundred thousand embryos are currently preserved frozen in the United States.

Since it is common to place more than one embryo at each attempt and since several of these may implant and develop, multiple-gestation pregnancies are a frequent consequence of IVF. This poses significant risks to the health of mother and fetuses. One solution to this problem is *selective reduction*, that is, the abortion of one or two of the multiple fetuses. We shall speak of this in topic 7 on abortion.

The technique of creating an embryo in vitro opens that embryo to direct observation and manipulation in the laboratory. It is possible to remove one or two cells from an embryo created in vitro and examine those cells for certain genetic characteristics. This technique, called *preimplantation genetic diagnosis* (PGD), is primarily intended to detect genetic defects so that an affected embryo can be discarded rather than implanted. Since the embryo is never implanted in the womb, the moral agony over abortion is avoided. Also, parents who wish to engender a child who can be an organ or tissue donor for an afflicted sibling may use PGD to determine compatibility. PGD also allows parents to discard an embryo whose gender does not match their desires. Since IVF involves some physical risk and entails use of resources, its use for gender selection has not been favored. Gender selection reinforces social stereotypes and may, as it has in some countries, such as India, seriously distort the ratio between men and woman in the society.

As PGD becomes more sophisticated, it will detect genetic defects for conditions that have a statistical probability of developing many years later, such as Alzheimer's disease, or conditions of variable seriousness, such as neurofibromatosis, which ranges from horrifying disfiguration to hardly noticeable discoloration of the skin. Also, PGD may become the means of genetically engineering desired characteristics into the fetus. If our knowledge of behavioral genetics advances, it may be possible to predict the risk of violent behavior or the prospect of certain talents. One author mentions "perfect pitch," a musical talent that is known to run in families: a husband and wife, both musicians, might want to assure that all their babies are "engineered" for a musical career. The question arises whether PGD should be used for these purposes.

Underlying many of the debates is a fundamental ethical question: should the field of ART be viewed according to the general principle of procreative liberty or a broader principle of social justice? This is the question raised by the ethicist in the glitzy magazine article cited at the beginning of this topic. The principle of procreative liberty sees decisions about procreation as quite private and rests heavily on the basic principle of autonomy. Persons have the moral right to generate children when and how they choose. In this light, most of the procedures and techniques of ART can be judged as ethically acceptable. The alternative view argues that procreative liberty fails to take seriously the familial and social values that surround reproduction. Injustices can be done to children, and situations of injustice can be caused when only the choices of the procreating parties are considered. Critics of procreative liberty believe that reproduction should be circumscribed by a strong philosophy of what it means to have a child, to raise a family, and to be responsible in society.

ART does pose serious question of social justice. Its procedures are very costly. Their fallibility often requires many repeat interventions. In the United States, most forms of ART are not covered by health insurance. It is estimated that some 1 million women each year could benefit from ART, while some 120,000 have access to it. As the story that opens this topic demonstrates, the benefits of ART flow largely to those able to pay its high costs. Even though less fortunate couples may have serious medical problems of infertility or may deeply desire a child, they will find this help beyond their means. On the other hand, if coverage is extended, the very personal and subjective needs that underlie the desire to reproduce may generate excessive use with excessive public costs.

Serious bioethical discussion of reproductive technologies continues. The questions, while raised by a remarkable new science and technology, are posed against a two-thousand-year-old tradition of sexual and reproductive morality within monogamous and procreative marriage. That paradigm, deeply impressed upon Western culture, makes the new questions seem either outrageous or challengingly problematic. The long-standing condemnation of abortion has left a legacy of concern about the moral standing of the fetus, complicating discussions about the "manipulation" of embryos that are now, as never before, available to be created, split, frozen, transferred, discarded, and experimented upon. A long-standing moral tradition tightly links coitus to conception and circumscribes coitus within the bonds of marriage. The unlinking of conception from coitus and from marriage continues to trouble the modern conscience, relaxed as it is about sexual morality.

These long traditions still sound loudly in some places. The Vatican issued a resounding condemnation of all reproductive technology as profoundly unnatural, regardless of intention.[5] In other places, the long tradition is more muted but can still be heard in restrictive views and legislation. Commercial surrogacy is outlawed in many jurisdictions. Commissions in several countries, such as Germany, France, and Italy, have recommended restrictive laws for ART. The Council of Europe established an international convention for the protection of human rights in genetics, reproductive technology, and other bioethical issues. English philosopher Jonathan Glover, who wrote the European Commission report on new reproductive technologies reflects, "The deep divisions over present developments are partly about whether they are in themselves acceptable. But partly they reflect concern that we may be sleepwalking, step by step, into a world which few of us would now choose."[6] One of the values of bioethical discourse is to keep the walkers awake as they trek into the future to which the reproductive and genetic sciences point.

NOTES

1. "Forever Fertile?" *San Francisco* (October 2003): 68–77.
2. G. Dustan, "Moral and Social Issues," in *Law and Ethics of AID and Embryo Transfer*, CIBA (Amsterdam/New York: Elsevier, 1973), 51.
3. Joseph Fletcher, *Ethics of Genetic Control: Ending Reproductive Roulette* (Garden City, NY: Anchor Press, 1974), 147
4. L. Kass, *Toward a More Natural Science: Biology and Human Affairs* (New York: Free Press, 1985), 43–79.
5. Congregation for the Doctrine of the Faith, *Instruction on Respect for Human Life in Its Origins and on the Dignity of Procreation* (Boston: St. Paul Press, 1987).
6. J. Glover, *Ethics of New Reproductive Technologies* (DeKalb: Northern Illinois University Press, 1989), 20.

BIBLIOGRAPHY

Alpern, K., ed. 1992. *The Ethics of Reproductive Technologies*. New York: Oxford University Press.
Cohen, C., ed. 1996. *New Ways of Making Babies: The Case of Egg Donation*. Bloomington: Indiana University Press.
Glover, J. 1989. *Ethics of New Reproductive Technologies*. The Glover Report to the European Commission. DeKalb: Northern Illinois University Press.
Harris, J., and S. Holm, eds. 1998. *The Future of Human Reproduction*. New York: Oxford University Press.
McGee, G. 2000. *The Perfect Baby: Parenthood in the New World of Cloning and Genetics*. Lanham, MD: Rowman & Littlefield.
Murray, T. 1996. *The Worth of a Child*. Berkeley: University of California Press.
President's Council on Bioethics. 2004. *Reproduction and Responsibility: The Regulation of New Biotechnologies*. Washington, DC: President's Council on Bioethics.

Reich, W., ed. 1995. "Reproductive Technologies," *Encyclopedia of Bioethics*. New York: Macmillan.

Robertson, J. 1994. *Children of Choice: Freedom and the New Reproductive Technologies*. Princeton, NJ: Princeton University Press.

Ryan, M. 2001. *The Ethics and Economics of Assisted Reproduction: The Cost of Longing*. Washington, DC: Georgetown University Press.

· *Topic 7* ·

Abortion

"Partial Birth Abortion Criminalized"

On November 7, 2003, President Bush signed a law forbidding doctors to perform a procedure called, politically, *partial birth abortion* and, medically, *intact dilatation and extraction*. This law, hotly debated and immediately contested in the courts, goes to the heart of the bitter American debate over abortion. Its central contention is that the procedure, performed in late pregnancy, involves "partially" delivering the fetus out of the uterus, then performing a procedure that will kill it. The medical definition is more precise: "a breech extraction of the [fetal] body except the head and partial evacuation of the intracranial contents of the living fetus to effect vaginal delivery of a dead but otherwise intact fetus."[1] Such a procedure may be used to terminate an advanced pregnancy, but it is unknown how often it is used (many obstetricians claim that it is hardly ever used). Since in Anglo-American jurisprudence, legal personhood begins with the delivery of the fetus out of the mother, the proponents of the law claim that the procedure is a "partial birth" and constitutes murder. Opponents of abortion prefer that any destruction of fetal life at any point in pregnancy be outlawed, but they believe this one procedure, rare as it may be, can convince lawmakers and the public that abortion is clearly murder. How are we to think about the ethics of abortion?

Abortion is a deeply divisive political issue in the United States. As a moral issue, it has a long history. As a personal decision, it wrenches the conscience of a woman who faces it. Ethicists have crafted philosophical arguments that try to articulate and refine the terms of the problem. Abortion is not only a significant moral issue in itself; it also involves theoretical questions, such as the personhood of the fetus, that have implications for many

77

other bioethical problems, as we shall see in topic 11, "Cloning and Stem Cell Research."

THE ETHICAL ARGUMENTS

Many women face the decision to end a pregnancy deliberately. Many reasons suggest such a decision: pregnancy results from intercourse outside marriage or by rape, the health of the mother is threatened, the fetus is affected by deformity or disease, an additional child would be an insupportable burden, or a baby is inconvenient or simply not desired. For many women, religious belief constrains their considerations since many faiths condemn abortion. From early centuries, the Catholic Church considered the abortion of a "formed fetus," that is, from about midway through pregnancy, a mortal sin; in the nineteenth century, abortion at any time after conception was forbidden. Many Protestant churches disapproved but did not wholly condemn abortion, although in recent years the evangelical churches have taken a stand much like that of Catholicism. While Judaism has no definitive prohibition, abortion compromised the pervasive Jewish duty to procreate. Abortion, whether strictly forbidden or reluctantly tolerated, has generally lived under a religious cloud. In most Western nations, up to the mid-twentieth century, a physician who performed an abortion committed a crime, and women who chose abortion were implicated in criminal activity. Thus, women who sought abortions were forced into secret, often dangerous, recourse to abortionists.

In the United States, laws that criminalized abortion were first passed in the mid-nineteenth century under the influence of the churches and with the strong support of physicians. Public debate over the legality of state statutes began in the 1920s, and in 1973, the U.S. Supreme Court determined that these state laws violated the implied constitutional right of privacy. The Court ruled that states could not prohibit a woman from obtaining an abortion until the time of fetal viability, the beginning of the seventh month of the pregnancy. Prior to viability, the decision about abortion was a matter for a woman and her doctor; the state could regulate the safety of abortions in the second trimester. After viability, a state could enact legislation prohibiting abortion, unless it was necessary to save the life or preserve the health of the mother (*Roe v. Wade*). This major legal decision, however, did not end the debate over the morality or even the legality of abortion in the United States. A vituperative, even violent, public debate raged around the issue. The Catholic Church strongly upheld its doctrinal position that human life begins at conception; thus, the fetus deserves full protection from its beginnings. Evangelical Protestants also joined in the campaign against abortion. Advocates of the right-to-life movement were pitted against the advocates of the right to choose.

The ethical claims about abortion range from the assertion that women have an absolute right over their own bodies and may decide whether or not they wish to host a fetus to the claim that the fetus has the full moral rights of a person from the instant of conception. Between these extremes lie many qualifications and distinctions that swing the argument in different directions. These arguments invoke a wide range of moral assumptions and a diversity of physiological, psychological, and social facts. The moral resolution of the question of abortion seems to many intractable.

Bioethicists were undeterred by this intractability. They undertook to articulate the arguments on both sides. Although it is assumed that opposition to abortion comes primarily from religious adherents, some theological bioethicists have found justifications for abortion. Joseph Fletcher sees it primarily as a matter of personal autonomy, thus as a woman's right to control her body. This right, he believes, trumps any presumptive claim on life that an as yet unborn entity had. The much more conservative Paul Ramsey builds his opposing argument on the theological premise that the sanctity of human life is ultimately grounded in the value God places on it. God spreads his protection over humankind: "before I formed thee in the womb, I knew thee. . . . I sanctified thee" (Jeremiah 1:5). Even with this strong affirmation of fetal value, Ramsey admits that a serious problem arises when one life is pitted against another, when the saving of the fetus imperils the mother or vice versa. He employs the ethical argument of double effect to analyze these situations: if an act entails two consequences, one morally desirable or obligatory, the other morally reprehensible, the act may be done if the morally reprehensible effect is an unintended consequence of achieving the morally desirable effect. Thus, it is the incapacitation of the fetus as a danger to the mother, not its direct killing, that is intended. Since one cannot be done without the other, the indirect taking of fetal life may be permitted to save maternal life. He even permits direct killing when both fetus and mother are in peril. Catholic moral theologians, who generally approve of double-effect arguments, explicitly reject them in the matter of abortion. They maintain that direct or indirect killing of a fetus is a serious moral wrong (except in the rare case where a surgical procedure to save the mother's life, such as excision of a cancerous uterus, also incidentally destroys a fetus).

Another pioneer of bioethics, Dan Callahan, criticized one-value solutions —both the Roman Catholic position that abortion is always wrong and the women's rights position that abortion is a matter of personal choice only— and urged a move toward a "very large and ambiguous middle ground" that he hopes will provide space for a public consensus on public policy and law. The middle ground is "a bias . . . in favor of protecting human life. . . . It is good, so far as humanly and morally possible, to favor and promote the preservation of human life." Callahan examines the arguments surrounding the beginning of human life. He finds the *developmental thesis*, a staged emergence of the fetus into moral standing, most convincing. In this view, the attribution of moral status evolves as the fetus matures (as I shall explain below). In this view, early abortion, for justifiable reasons, is morally licit. Callahan believes that abortion decisions should be left to the women themselves, but public policy should be designed to promote the protection of unborn life by many means: liberal availability of contraception, social alternatives to abortion, counseling, and education.[2]

Philosopher Judith Thomson has formulated an argument in support of abortion in an article frequently reprinted in ethics textbooks. She imagines a bizarre case: a woman awakens to find that a famous, dying violinist is hooked to her body and only by remaining hooked can he continue to live. He claims a right to the woman's body. Is it morally right to unhook him? Thomson then draws an analogy with the fetus, hooked up to a woman's body for life support: just as you can unhook the violinist intruding on your body, so a woman can disconnect the fetus. Thomson is not asserting that the attached being is harming the woman (many traditional arguments in favor of abortion turn on whether the fetal presence or birth is dangerous to the mother); she simply argues that the woman does not want or have any obligation to serve in this way. Thomson's argument aims to justify the claim that the abortion decision turns entirely on the moral right of a woman to control her body.

If the abortion debate pits a woman's right to choose against the fetus's right to life, the contentious question about the moral status of the fetus must be addressed. Does that maternal right to choose confront any fetal right to exist? Certainly, the chromosomes and genes involved in the making of an embryo belong to the genetic species that is human. But the word "human" does not have only a genetic meaning. It also designates a kind of being that is to be valued and treated in certain ways. We must ask whether this genetically human being is also to be counted among the class of moral beings called human. Where in the universe of living things, plants, animals, and humans does the embryo belong? The question has been asked since antiquity. Orthodox Jews cite biblical texts of great antiquity that refer to the early embryo as "like water" and impart to it no special moral status. Ancient biologists, such as Aristotle, believed that an embryo begins life as a vegetable, develops into an animal, then, when all organs are formed, into a human being. The embryo certainly does not look very human: it starts life rather plantlike in cellular structure, and as it assumes shape, it looks as much like a mouse as a human. Only at the end of the first trimester does it begin to look like a baby and is its name changed to fetus.

This developing appearance is driven by a genetic program, originating in the parental DNA joined at fertilization. Thus, the first plausible answer to the question of moral status could be that at the instant two human genetic packages join into one (approximately when the head of a sperm penetrates the nucleus of an ovum, each carrying a package of twenty-three chromosomes and uniting in a zygote with forty-six chromosomes), a human person is generated. At that moment, the full responsibilities that obtain between human persons are also generated. This is the position taken by the Roman Catholic Church. "From the moment of conception," says the Vatican document *Gift of Life*, "the life of every human being is to be respected in an absolute way. . . . Human life is sacred because from its beginning it involves the 'creative action of God.' . . . [N]o one can, in any circumstance, claim for himself the right to destroy directly an innocent human being."[3] Many other religious faiths take this position. Even some persons who are not religiously affiliated consider it a plausible position: after all, we all begin life as a fertilized ovum, and the genetic program that forms us is human from the beginning.

Another response to the moral question relies not on the genetic origins of the embryo but on its staged progress from zygote to baby. There are many milestones in that progress. It makes sense, say those who hold this position, to attribute moral personhood to the fetus only as it reaches certain of those milestones. Implantation in the womb occurs at about six days after fertilization; at about fourteen days, the formation of the primitive streak sets embryo on its way to individuality. Up to that time, the embryo (some call it the preembryo) is a ball, then a flat sheet of undifferentiated cells. Then, the sheet begins to fold, a centerline appears, genes that make cells specific, such as neurons and tissue, turn on, and organs begin to form. At this point, the embryo can no longer split into twins.

Many commentators see the primitive streak as a significant marker of human personhood. Moral obligations can be ascribed only when individuation has taken place, for only then can it be said that the developing entity is at the start of being a person. Some proponents of this view claim that at this point in development, the fetus acquires the absolute rights of moral personhood. Others maintain that as the fetus develops physically, increasingly stringent moral restrictions should be placed on how the fetus is treated. Adherents of this view do not oppose destruction of an embryo or its use for research up to fourteen days of life, when the primitive streak appears. The Australian Commission, the British Warnock Report, and the American Ethics Advisory Board documents mentioned in topic 6 take this position. Other points in fetal development impress some ethicists as crucial for the attribution of personhood. The emergence of neurological activity at about two months of gestation, a sort of "brain birth" by analogy with "brain death," has won some adherents.

A final position maintains that only when the fetus has a firm enough hold on existence that it can live independently of its mother do significant moral duties toward it appear. In this view, viability, the time at which organ systems, particularly the lungs, can function, even with artificial support, is the most suitable milestone at which to attribute moral personhood. This is the position taken by the U.S. Supreme Court in *Roe v. Wade*. The position of Orthodox Judaism goes even beyond viability: the actual birth of a child begins its personhood and entitlement to rights. Abortion up to that point is permissible (although rabbis surround that permissibility with many fences).

Bioethicists have debated these complex questions about the beginning of personhood, the definition of personal identity, and the relevance of viability as a marker for the protection of fetal life. Despite sophisticated arguments, the debate always resolves into the poles of the fetus's right to life (whenever defined) and the mother's right to choose. In that form, shorn of most philosophical niceties, the debate stands as a matter for public contention and political dispute. However, even those who argue in favor of abortion in principle may be troubled by the reasons why some women choose abortion.

Proponents of the absolute right to choose abortion, based on the principle of autonomy, do not quibble about reasons. Yet, abortion as a means of family planning, when so many other options are available, troubles some. Even more, abortion in order to obtain a child of a desired sex meets with moral disfavor among many otherwise permissive ethicists. This practice has implications for equality among the sexes and for population balance: its use in India, for example, has led to a notable imbalance between men and women. The ability to diagnose whether the fetus has a medical or genetic problem began with the introduction of amniocentesis in the 1970s and now has moved to the technique of preimplantation genetic diagnosis mentioned in topic 6. Diagnostic and screening tests for some four hundred conditions of considerable variability are currently available. Parents may consider abortion the tragic consequence of a prenatal diagnosis of serious fetal anomaly. Yet, this practice forces conscientious people to reflect on the meaning of disability and its impact on those affected, their families, and society. Some ethicists have cautioned that the practice of destroying disabled fetal life depreciates the living disabled. It may also depreciate our compassion and altruism.

ART has presented a new form of the abortion problem. Since ART not infrequently leads to multiple-gestation pregnancies (twins or triplets or more) and since multiple-gestation pregnancies pose significant threats to the health of mother and fetuses, it is sometimes recommended that one or several of the fetuses be terminated in order to reduce the risks to the survivor(s). This *selective reduction* is a unique form of the abortion dilemma. Presumably, parents want these babies; all fetuses in the multiple gestation are wanted. One or several of the fetuses poses a threat to its siblings. An ethicist opposed to abortion simply would find no justification for selective reduction. However, an ethicist opposed to abortion generally but not universally might find a self-defense justification. However, even then, it would not be clear in most cases which fetus is the aggressor and why. The "aggressor" is selected somewhat at random (and is often the smallest fetus). Indeed, can mere coexistence in the same womb count as aggression? Also, the procedures used to selectively reduce the embryos are themselves risky, increasing the risk of miscarriage and infection, so that an attempt to aid the survivor may lead to its mortality or morbidity. Selective reduction is truly an ethical paradox.

Abortion is an ancient moral problem. However, the contemporary debate over abortion, both philosophical and political, has a very modern feature. It poses the very modern value of personal autonomy, interpreted as a major moral principle, against the traditional moral injunction prohibiting the taking of life. In that form, it parallels many other bioethical issues, such as those concerning the end of life that we saw in the opening topics.

NOTES

1. American College of Obstetrics and Gynecology, *Statement on Intact Dilatation and Extraction*, January 12, 1997.
2. D. Callahan, *Abortion: Law, Choice and Morality* (New York: Macmillan, 1970), 19, 495.
3. Sacred Congregation for the Doctrine of the Faith, *Donum Vitae* (Vatican City: 1987).

BIBLIOGRAPHY

Brody, B. 1975. *Abortion and the Sanctity of Life*. Cambridge, MA: MIT Press.
Callahan, D. 1970. *Abortion: Law, Choice and Morality*. New York: Macmillan.
Dworkin, R. *Life's Dominion: An Argument about Abortion, Euthanasia and Individual Freedom*. New York: Knopf.
Feinberg, J., ed. 1973. *The Problem of Abortion*. Belmont, CA: Wadsworth Publishing.

Hauerwas, S. 1990. *Naming the Silences: God, Medicine and the Problem of Suffering.* Grand Rapids, MI: Eerdmans.

Kamm, F. 1992. *Creation and Abortion: A Study in Moral and Legal Philosophy.* New York: Oxford University Press.

Noonan, J., ed. 1970. *The Morality of Abortion: Legal and Historical Perspectives.* Cambridge, MA: Harvard University Press.

Reich, W., ed. 1995. "Abortion," *Encyclopedia of Bioethics.* New York: Macmillan.

Sumner, L. 1981. *Abortion and Moral Theory.* Princeton, NJ: Princeton University Press.

III

SCIENTIFIC BIOETHICS: THE SEARCH FOR BENEFIT

*T*he topics of part II dealt with bioethical problems that arise when patients and physicians encounter in clinical settings. Part III moves to the scientific world that surrounds clinical medicine. In clinical medicine the essential task is to cure the patient. In scientific medicine the essential task is to discover new and better forms of treatment. Medicial scientists glimpse these possibilities and attempt to make them real by experiments in the laboratory and in the clinic. In this world, many of the ethical problems look to the future: they are of the "what if we could" sort. The prospects excite us and trouble us. It must be noted, however, that since all of these sciences have already reached into clinical care, some of the problems we discuss are already with us as clinical ethical problems. Many other problems, however, exist in anticipation as scientists make the future real bit by bit. Often, the media will excite us about some "ethical problem" that is, in reality, still distant. Its distance, however, is no reason not to think seriously about it.

· *Topic 8* ·

Research with Humans: Experimentation, Autonomy, and Benefits to Others

"Boy in Medical Experiment Dies"

*E*ighteen-year-old Jesse Gelsinger had a rare genetic disease, ornithine car-bamylase deficiency, a liver disease caused by a gene mutation. Although fatal in itself, this disease can sometimes be rather mild. Jesse had a mild form, alleviated by medication and diet. Scientists had identified the genetic mutation that causes the disease and were hoping to develop a genetic therapy, in which inserting a normal gene would correct the metabolic disorder. They sought volunteers for an experiment. Jesse learned about the project and volunteered. He knew that the research was only an early step, would probably not benefit him, but might relieve many future sufferers. He traveled to the University of Pennsylvania, where researchers injected his body with an adenovirus (the germ involved in the common cold) into which a copy of the normal gene had been engineered. A few hours after the injection, Jesse became acutely ill. Three days later, he died. An investigation revealed that the researchers had failed to report two previous cases of liver toxicity following the injection and, thus, had failed to include that information in the informed consent that Jesse was given on admission to the study. Also, a serious conflict of interest on the part of the chief scientist, Dr. James Wilson, raised questions about his motives in concealing the negative effects. He was an investor in and scientific advisor to the company that was sponsoring the research. The tragedy of Jesse Gelsinger's death prompted a reevaluation of gene therapy, as well as a searching review of the system of research ethics and regulation that had long been relied upon to prevent such tragedies.

Every clinical activity, even in the most straightforward medicine, has margins of uncertainty. Bioscience constitutes a deliberate and structured

86

rational activity to dispel that uncertainty and to discover effective forms of medical treatment. As bioethics moves from clinical medicine into the world of the biosciences, the familiar moral grounding of the interpersonal relationship between patients and doctors begins to fade. New forms of ethical perplexity appear in which the ethics built around the injunction to "be of benefit and do no harm" are only a partial guide. The compelling vision of improved health in a better society requires a more elaborate interplay between the principles of bioethics. Does a search for future good override individual liberty or safety? Is justice to future generations more imperative than obligations to the living generation? Under what ethical provisions may scientists put persons at risk not for their benefit but to expand knowledge? The topic of experimentation raises these questions.

The word "experimentation" comes from the Latin word for "experience." In the past, doctors tried various treatments and, by experience, found that some of them seemed to remedy ailments. But "seemed to" was the problem: is it possible to prove that certain medicines or maneuvers do more good than harm? Beginning in the nineteenth century, experimentation evolved into research, a systematic search for proven, generalizable knowledge about diseases and treatments. It was performed in clinics with patients and in laboratories with healthy persons, often the researchers themselves. Its ethical implications were seldom noticed. However, medical experimentation burst into the consciousness of the public when, in 1947, the Nuremberg War Crimes Tribunal sentenced to imprisonment and death a group of Nazi medical scientists who had performed mutilating, often lethal, experiments on prisoners in concentration camps. The Nuremberg Code, formulated at the Nuremberg Trial, became a universally acknowledged statement of the ethics of research with humans. Its first principle states,

> The voluntary consent of the human subject is absolutely essential. This means that the person involved should have legal capacity to give consent; should be so situated as to be able to exercise free power of choice[;] . . . and should have sufficient knowledge and comprehension of the elements of the subject matter involved as to enable him to make an understanding and enlightened decision. . . . [B]efore the acceptance of an affirmative decision by the experimental subject there should be made known to him the nature, duration and purpose of the experiment; the method and means by which it is to be conducted; all inconveniences and hazards reasonably to be expected; and their effects upon his health or person which may possibly come from his participation in the experiment.[1]

The formal legal words veil the horror of the concentration camps in which these "experimental subjects," totally stripped of their freedom and dignity, were mutilated and murdered under the guise of scientific research. The code's second principle, that "the experiment should be such as to yield fruitful results for the good of society," directs research to a human good rather than to the goals of an ideology. The code's other principles require prior experiments with animals, avoidance of unnecessary physical and mental suffering and injury, a priori assurance that no death or disabling injury will result, use of scientifically qualified researchers, and guarantees of the subject's right and the researcher's duty to terminate harmful experiments. Another major statement of research ethics, the Helsinki Declaration (1954), was issued by the World Medical Association.

These statements of principle contrasted sharply with several highly publicized events in the United States. At Willowbrook State Hospital in New York, mentally retarded children were infected with hepatitis in order to study the natural history of that disease and to seek a vaccine against it. At Jewish Chronic Disease Hospital in Brooklyn, elderly demented patients were injected with cancer cells. The July 26, 1972, edition of the *New York Times* carried a shocking story: "For forty years, the United States Public Health Service has conducted a study in which human beings with syphilis, who were induced to serve as guinea pigs, have gone without treatment for the disease. . . . [T]he study was conducted to determine from autopsies what the disease does to the human body." The subjects of the study were "about 600 black men, mostly poor and uneducated, from Tuskegee, Alabama." The men had been promised free transportation to and from hospitals, free hot lunches, free medical care for any disease other than syphilis, and free burial after autopsies were performed.[2]

In the next days and weeks, details of the Tuskegee study were revealed in the press. Of the six hundred research subjects, four hundred had been diagnosed with syphilis but were never told and never treated. The other two hundred who did not have syphilis were "controls." None were ever informed that they were research subjects or that treatment for their condition could have been provided. Patients and controls alike were told that they had "bad blood" and should have periodic medical examinations, including annual spinal taps. In 1972, when the study was officially closed, seventy-four of the untreated subjects were still living. A federal panel examined the program, severely criticized its design and implementation, and suggested oversight of federally funded research. The few survivors were modestly compensated. Years later, President Clinton publicly apologized to them and to all touched by this misguided project.

The public exposure of these events aroused concern about research, an enterprise most people had seen as unequivocally beneficial. People were vividly aware that medicine was improving rapidly due to scientific progress, and the U.S. Congress was pouring millions into the National Institutes of Health for the promotion of research. They could hardly imagine that this progress was associated with abuse of human subjects. A few scientists and physicians, such as Henry Beecher in the United States and M. H. Pappworth in Britain, began to criticize the prevailing ethics of research.

THE ETHICAL ARGUMENTS

Research searches for a future, common good. This scientific endeavor seems to fit perfectly into the ethical theory of *utilitarianism*. This theory, widely accepted within Anglo-American philosophy and seeming so sensible to many educated persons, maintains that any action should be judged as morally right if and only if it tends to produce the greater good for the greater number. Research is an endeavor specifically designed to produce greater good for the greater number. Does this goal justify "using" individuals to produce these goods? In the past, many researchers strongly believed that it did. A leading American physician once stated, "The core of this ethical issue [is] to ensure the rights of society [to new treatments], even if an arbitrary judgment must be made against an individual." Society gains its right over individuals, he proposed, "from the demonstration that knowledge gained by studies in a few humans can show us how to operate programs of great practical benefit to the group. . . . Society, too, has rights in human experimentation. We will have to learn how to institutionalize 'playing god,' while maintaining the key elements of a free society."[3]

However, the research subject is a human being, not a guinea pig. It is ethically necessary to ask whether research subjects can be treated merely as a means to attain an end foreign to their own welfare. The German philosopher Immanuel Kant famously stated that "the supreme practical principle or . . . categorical imperative . . . [is to] act in such a way that you always treat humanity, whether in your own person or in the person of any other, never simply as a means, but always at the same time as an end."[4] This is Kant's version of the principle of autonomy. In part I, I noted the centrality of respect for autonomy in bioethics and explained this principle as an implication of John Stuart Mill's basic thesis about liberty: no one is entitled to interfere in the actions or choices of others except to prevent them from harming others. In the ethics of research, the Kantian meaning of autonomy rather than the Millsian one is dominant. Research on a human being, conducted in order to draw from that person knowledge for the treatment of others or for the profit of the researcher, appears a clear case of using that person as "simply a means."

The ethics of research, then, becomes a face-off between arguments reflecting two powerful ethical theories, Kantianism and utilitarianism. Does the prohibition against using persons as a means obstruct the pursuit of the greater good for the greater number? Does the greater good justify exposing persons to risk? The Kantian stricture may be overcome only if the person becomes a volunteer. Thus, the first move in elaborating an ethics of research was to stress the importance of free and informed consent to serve as a research subject. The participant must not only be educated about the nature of the research, its risks, and, in particular, its objective to benefit future patients and the progress of medicine, but he or she must enter the research as a willing collaborator. The face-off between Kantian research ethics and utilitarian research ethics is eased: it is ethical to pursue the common good of new knowledge through the use of human participants but only if those persons consent to be used. This ethic, of course, was utterly violated by the Nazi doctors and by the American scientists at Tuskegee.

The ethical dimensions of research are not limited to the consent of the subject. The scientific design of the research study also poses serious ethical questions. As medical research gained in momentum, methods of research became more elaborate and formal. Today, researchers no longer simply perform some tests and report what appeared to be their results. Rather, specific designs to compare data and overcome observer bias have been designed; sophisticated statistical mathematics analyze the results. The *controlled clinical trial*, using techniques such as randomization of subjects between treatments and placebos and the "blinding" of researcher and subject to the nature of the intervention, has vastly improved the confidence that researchers, physicians and the public can place in research results.

These methods themselves have raised significant ethical problems. British statistician Sir Bradford Hill, a pioneer of research design, noted the main ethical problems of the controlled clinical trial: determination of the safety of the proposed intervention, the relative values of old and new treatment, the random allocation of patients to different arms of the trial, the patient's consent, placebos, and blinding of physician to the treatment being administered. In order to initiate an ethically valid research study, the researcher must make a sound judgment, based on clinical experience and prior studies, that the current treatments and the test treatment are at least equivalent in risks and benefits. The researcher's task is to prove that the test treatment is superior. No one should be able to affirm, prior to the conclusion of the research, whether a person receiving the standard treatment or the test treatment (or placebo) is better off. This judgment came to be known as *clinical equipoise*.[5] This equipoise is extraordinarily difficult to determine, requiring an extensive and exquisite analysis of data; yet, it is a key ingredient in evaluating the research methods.

Philosopher Hans Jonas made a landmark contribution to the ethics of research in "Philosophical Reflections on Experimenting with Human Subjects." Jonas acknowledges that the most common way of conceptualizing the moral problem of research sees a polarity between the good of individuals and the common good. He denies that this is the proper way to frame the problem. Rights and obligations are moral concepts that center on the protection of society from disintegration and of individuals from harm. It is claimed, he notes, that experimentation is justified by the common good of society. But experimentation, by its very nature, produces the good not of preservation of social life but of progress and enhancement. These goals are *melioristic* (*melior* is Latin for "better," thus, making better) and are not obligatory: "our descendants have a right to be left an unplundered planet; they do not have a right to new miracle cures." The pursuit of melioristic goals cannot generate any "right" of society over the "right" of the individual. Melioristic goals, while not obligatory, are noble: they call humans to a free, even sacrificial, engagement of self. The social enterprise of experimentation must be seen within "an ethical dimension [that] far exceeds that of the moral law and reaches into the sublime solitude of dedication and ultimate commitment."[6]

Jonas brings this vision to medical experimentation. Consent is not enough. True volunteering, that is, active engagement in the purposes of another and identifying them with one's own purposes, is the proper justification for research. He suggests that the persons most identified with the melioristic goal, the researchers themselves, should be the first volunteers (as they often were in the early days of experimental medicine). Those poorer in knowledge, motivation, and freedom of decision, such as children, the developmentally disabled, and persons with psychiatric conditions, should be the last. These latter candidates are not absolutely excluded, but more compelling reasons must justify approaching them. In this light, "Human experimentation . . . involves ultimate questions of personal dignity and sacrosancitity."

While Jonas's essay dwells in the thin air of "philosophical reflections," its principal proposition is a powerfully compelling one: participation in research must be seen, in all its aspects and for all participants, as an exercise in freedom. Society cannot infringe on individual rights for the production of its future goods. It cannot physically or by deception "conscript" persons into research. Further, research subjects are generally highly vulnerable. Often, they suffer from the disease that is under study and cannot easily distinguish between the therapy they need and the scientific knowledge that the researchers seek. Research subjects may not be able to comprehend either the research procedures or the idea of research as essentially voluntary. They may be awed by the prestige of the researcher or of the institution. Researchers must be aware of all this and take measures to correct the obstacles to true voluntariness.

PUBLIC POLICY ABOUT RESEARCH ETHICS

In the wake of the Tuskegee experiments and other abuses, Congress established the National Commission for the Protection of Human Subjects of Biomedical and Behavioral Research (1974–1978). The commission was to study how best to protect the rights and welfare of research subjects in projects funded by the federal government (at that time, the major supporter of biomedical research). The commission issued the Belmont Report (1978), a document that became the central declaration of research ethics in the United States.[7]

The Belmont Report states three basic ethical principles that should govern research with humans: respect for persons, beneficence and nonmaleficence, and justice. Respect for persons incorporates two ethical convictions: first, that individuals should be treated as autonomous agents, and second, that persons with diminished autonomy are entitled to protection. The practical application of this principle requires adequate informed consent to participate in research. Beneficence requires promoting the well-being of research subjects. This principle requires a careful assessment of the risks and benefits of the research not only to the subject but to medical science and to society. Justice requires a fair distribution of the benefits and burdens of research. This principle requires that research subjects be selected in an equitable manner and that the burdens and risks of research not fall unduly on a certain class or group.

The commission endorsed the establishment of institutional review boards (IRBs) in all research institutions. These IRBs discuss research not in the abstract but in the concrete particulars of specific protocols. Reviewers inspect the protocols submitted to them, seeking the rationale for the research, the justification for using human subjects, the risks and benefits to the subjects, and the expression of all this in an accurate consent form. Reviewers may send the protocol back to its authors for improvement and, if ultimately dissatisfied, can reject it. Rejection means that the project will not be funded (review is obligatory for all research, regardless of the source of funding). The federal government established the IRB system, which has functioned with considerable success for several decades. In the United Kingdom, the Department of Health recommended that all research institutions establish research ethics committees (RECs) with similar purposes. While in both nations research institutions are responsible for vetting research, government agencies provide considerable oversight and guidance. These systems of regulation and oversight have provided several decades of research free of the scandals that inspired them. In the 1990s, however, cracks in the system began to appear. The case of Jesse Gelsinger revealed one of those cracks.

In the current system, consent of the subject and design of the research protocol are central to research ethics. Jesse was not adequately informed. However, a third major problem of research ethics appeared in the Gelsinger case: conflict of interest. Ironically, it had long been noted that when physicians become researchers, they take a different moral stance toward a patient, moving from exclusive caregiver to scientific investigator. These two roles may seriously conflict. However, concern over this conflict of interest rarely found its way into bioethical debate or public policy until the 1990s. Significant shifts from government to commercial funding of research introduced the possibility of profit into scientific investigations: scientists could become shareholders in companies that sponsored their work. The incentive for putting subjects at risk and of distorting data, always present for fame, now become more serious for fortune. Jesse Gelsinger's investigator was an investor in the gene therapy company.

Questions continue to haunt research ethics. The controlled clinical trial remains the paradigm for research, but its scientific rigidity has made it difficult to gain data on rare conditions, which become *orphan diseases* without effective treatment. High costs of controlled trials discourage companies from research on diseases where an effective therapy might be less profitable. The therapeutic equipoise that justifies research testing of a current therapy against an investigative one can easily tip into *therapeutic misconception*, namely, the misconception that the investigative treatment is in fact effective, particularly when it is seen as a last chance. It has also become clear that research design formerly systematically excluded women (due to fear of damaging fetal life) and that drugs used for pediatric conditions had not been tested in children. These two excluded classes of research subjects now must be added to those to whom the principle of justice in research must be applied. Treatment of persons with compromised mental capacity has been hindered; their mental incapacity often precludes informed consent, making it difficult to design protocols that can ethically include them, although research into their treatment is urgently needed.

Research in genetics enters into the issue of personal privacy more deeply than most biomedical research. Research involving whole communities of persons, particularly those with unique cultural heritages, must respect the customs of those groups. Research done abroad, particularly in developing nations, must both respect local norms and adhere to American standards, which are often difficult to apply in quite different cultures. Informed consent, for example, may make little sense in a culture where group consensus or the permission of a chief prevails. There is also concern about exploitation of vulnerable populations. It is now asserted that if a new drug or treatment is developed by using inhabitants of a developing country as subjects, the new product should be made "reasonably available" to those who undertook the risks of its development. As the world confronts bioterrorism, experiments to protect whole societies against lethal agents are imperative; yet, designing such studies, which also respect the rights of individuals, is problematic. Finally, in a dramatic reversal of concept, some persons do not wish to be "protected" from research: they desire to be included when they see research as the only promise of relief from their conditions. They demand admission to trials, although they may not meet scientific criteria for inclusion.

Research ethics is a highly developed part of bioethics. It works with a set of clearly defined ethical concepts. Its mark is seen in regulation and review of research by oversight bodies in most countries. At the same time, the tension remains between the deontological arguments flowing from respect for individuals and the utilitarian arguments flowing from common future goods. Many practical problems of implementing even the best regulations also remain. New forms of research challenge traditional concepts. Research is a search for benefits as yet unrealized: it must be undertaken with high sensitivity not only to risks but to the generous autonomy of volunteers.

NOTES

1. *Trials of War Criminals before the Nuremberg Military Tribunals* (Washington, DC: U.S. Government Printing Office, 1949), II:181, in *Source Book in Bioethics*, ed. A. Jonsen, R. Veatch, and L. Walters (Washington, DC: Georgetown University Press), 11.

2. "Syphilis Victims in US Study Went Untreated for 40 Years," *New York Times*, July 26, 1972, A1, A8.

3. W. McDermott, cited in A. Jonsen, *The Birth of Bioethics* (New York: Oxford University Press, 1998), 164.

4. I. Kant, *Groundwork of the Metaphysic of Morals*, trans. H. Paton (New York: Harper Torchbooks, 1964), ch. 2, 66, 96.

5. B. Freedman, "Equipoise and the Ethics of Clinical Trials," *New England Journal of Medicine* 327 (1987): 141–45.

6. Hans Jonas, "Philosophical Reflections on Experimenting with Human Subjects," *Daedalus* 98 (1969): 219–47, 230.

7. National Commission for the Protection of Human Subjects of Biomedical and Behavioral Research, *The Belmont Report: Ethical Principles and Guidelines for the Protection of Human Subjects in Research*, in *Source Book in Bioethics*, A. Jonsen, R. Veatch, and L. Walters, 22.

BIBLIOGRAPHY

Advisory Committee on Human Radiation Experiments. 1996. *The Human Radiation Experiments.* New York: Oxford University Press.

Beauchamp, T., and J. Childress. 1991. *Principles of Biomedical Ethics*, ch. 7. New York: Oxford University Press.

Beecher, H. 1970. *Research and the Individual.* Boston: Little, Brown and Company.

Brody, B. 2001. *The Ethics of Biomedical Research: An International Perspective.* New York: Oxford University Press.

Jones, J. 1981. *Bad Blood.* New York: Free Press.

Jonsen, A. 1998. *The Birth of Bioethics,* ch. 5. New York: Oxford University Press.

Kahn, J., A. Mastroianni, and J. Sugarman. 1998. *Beyond Consent: Seeking Justice in Research.* New York: Oxford University Press.

Levine, R. 1988. *Ethics and Regulation of Clinical Research.* New Haven, CT: Yale University Press.

Moreno, J. 2001. *Undue Risk: Secret State Experiments on Humans.* New York: Routledge.

National Bioethics Advisory Commission. 2001. *Ethical and Policy Issues in Research Involving Human Participants.* Springfield, VA: U.S. Department of Commerce, at www.bioethics.georgetown.edu/nbac.

National Commission for the Protection of Human Subjects. 1998. *Source Book in Bioethics,* ed. A. Jonsen, R. Veatch, and L. Walters. Washington, DC: Georgetown University Press.

Pappworth, M. 1968. *Human Guinea Pigs: Experimentation in Medicine.* New York: Beacon Press.

Reich, W. 1995. "Research, Human," *Encyclopedia of Bioethics.* New York: Macmillan.

Genetics

"Fatal Disease Gene Discovered"

$\mathcal{D}$r. Nancy Wexler has done pioneering work in finding the gene that causes the devastating disease called Huntington's chorea. This neurological condition destroys first the ability to walk and control movement, then demolishes the mind, leading to fifteen or twenty years of convulsive, demented life before death. It has long been known that this terrible disease is inherited: if only one parent has it, every child has a 50 percent chance of inheriting it. Dr. Wexler's interest is more than scientific: her mother died of Huntington's disease. As she has worked over the years with populations of patients afflicted or threatened, she knows that she too could become a victim. Now that she and her scientific colleagues have identified the gene and tests are available that can confirm that a person carries it, Dr. Wexler has decided not to have the test.

Jane K. was diagnosed with breast cancer when she was fifty-one years old. She underwent a mastectomy with radiation. She suspects that breast cancer may be hereditary in her family. She knows that her aunt died of breast cancer and suspects that her grandmother did as well. Jane has two adult sisters, two daughters, ages twenty-three and seventeen, and one granddaughter, age two. She has read that genetic tests for two forms of inheritable breast cancer are available: these tests detect mutations in two genes, designated as BRCA 1 and BRCA 2. She wonders whether she, her sisters, her daughters, and grandchild should be tested. She, of course, has already had cancer, but would a positive test predict future cancer in her relatives?

Dr. Wexler and Ms. K. are in the world of genetic medicine. In the last decade, many tests have been devised to locate gene mutations associated with a variety of diseases. In traditional medicine, disease is suspected when persons experience symptoms, such as pain, nausea, weakness; genetic medicine predicts a potential for disease before symptoms appear (although genetic tests may also confirm a physical diagnosis or provide added information). Neither Dr. Wexler's nor Ms. K.'s relatives have any symptoms of disease (and may never have). Tests can be given to a couple before marriage to detect whether either or both carry harmful genes that might affect their offspring. Tests can be applied to the fetus in the womb and even to an embryo created in the laboratory and not yet implanted in a womb to determine the risk of genetic disease. An individual can be tested to determine risk of a future disease.

Unlike most medical information, genetic information is not only about the patient tested. It may also tell a story about that patient's kin, for genetic information is usually about the genes shared between blood relatives and those who marry them. Genetic testing is already part of clinical practice: cases like that of Dr. Wexler and Jane K., as well as many other more complex ones, are not uncommon. They raise ethical issues about how information is gained and imparted, how it should be used, and how that information, often intensely personal, should be guarded with the confidentiality customary in medicine. This topic reviews some of these questions. It then discusses ethical problems that lie in the future, for they attach to practices that remain in the imagination of scientists, in laboratory dishes, and to some extent, in clinical experimentation, as was the case with Jesse Gelsinger. Some of the most troubling ethical issues are about the future, rather than present, capabilities of genetic science. One geneticist coined the word "genethics" to name this set of issues.[1]

GENETIC SCIENCE

The science of genetics flourished during the twentieth century. The theory of inheritable factors, first called *genes* about the beginning of the century, began with natural observation of inherited traits in plants, insects, animals, and people and was transformed into science by the statistical rules stated by Abbot Mendel (published first in the mid-nineteenth century, then lost to view until rediscovered in 1900). Genetics was propelled into a laboratory science soon thereafter by scientists studying the inherited patterns of insects, and after World War II, an extraordinary collaboration of biologists, chemists, physicists, and statisticians transformed it by application of chemical and physical techniques. The science of molecular biology, which explored cells and chromosomes, opened up the vast complexity and the elegant structure of the inheritable factor, which was recognized as deoxyribonucleic acid (DNA), the main constituent of the chromosomes that exist and work in almost every cell of every organism.

In 1953, Francis Crick and James Watson at Cambridge University gave scientists a clear picture of the structure and function of DNA as a *double helix*, two intertwined strands built from four chemical bases. Those bases arranged in different order carry the information that eventually results in the proteins that make up the body's every organ and tissue. The twining and untwining of the strands sets off the process whereby cells proliferate, and the genetic structure is passed on to new organisms (usually) in sexual reproduction. Long segments of these strands make up *genes*, sequences of DNA that send out chemical information, a code that the organism can read to build itself, make itself function, and replicate itself in progeny.

There are forty-six chromosomes in almost every cell of the human body. On each chromosome, there are millions of base pairs; those base pairs sort out into approximately twenty thousand genes (at latest count). Modifications and defects in those sequences, such as omission or excessive repetition or mix-up of bases, can set off the processes that cause disease. For example, a series of bases on chromosome 4, usually repeated about fifteen times, can expand, with the effect of producing an excess of a particular protein that can clog and destroy neural cells: this is the cause of the dreaded Huntington's disease. Sometimes defective genes need only be inherited from one parent, as in Huntington's disease; for most single-gene diseases, the defect must come from the joining of two defective genes, one from each parent. The scientific reading of genes can be translated into information for patients and parents so that they may make decisions about their futures and future children. As genetics becomes an information science, its impact on human life goes far beyond the physical: it deeply affects personal and social life. Indeed, some scientists have became fond of speaking of the genetic code as the writing in the Book of Life.

The science of molecular genetics unfolded so rapidly after the structure of DNA was elucidated that the idea of identifying the exact location of genes on chromosomes and specifying their chemical makeup—or mapping and sequencing the human genome—quickly leapt to the scientific mind. This idea was transformed into a research reality, sponsored by the U.S. government as the Human Genome Project. A first draft of the human genome was completed in the late 1990s, opening vast research possibilities and bringing scientific genetics closer to clinical medicine.

Dr. Watson, leader of the Human Genome Project, realized that it was not only a major advance in biology but also an ethical minefield. He was prudent enough to see that by adding an ethics component to the scientific study, he would assuage some of those concerns. He set aside 3 to 5 percent of the project's budget for research into the ethical, legal, and social implications of the scientific project (the ELSI program). It was important to be clear about the ways in which genetic information about individuals and populations would be used clinically, commercially, and politically. How would confidentiality be protected? How would diseases that affected particular populations be studied without stigmatizing those populations and endangering their reputations, livelihood, and insurability?

GENETIC DIAGNOSIS AND TESTING

Genetic diagnosis and testing means many things. It can refer to *risk assessment*, tracing a disease through a family tree and calculating the probability that the person being tested might have inherited the gene that contributes to that disease and how likely it is that he or she will pass it on. This form of genetic assessment was possible prior to the explosion of molecular genetics: it relies only on family interviews, family histories of disease, and statistical analysis of patterns of inheritance. Genetic testing may also entail biochemical tests of blood or tissue that reveal the presence or absence of some enzyme known to be harmful. For example, a simple blood test can reveal high levels of phenylalanine, which, if undetected, can cause phenylketonuria (PKU). Abnormal levels of phenylalanine result from a gene mutation that is inherited as recessive; that is, the child must receive one copy of the mutated gene from each parent. Babies appear normal for months after birth, then begin to show signs of developmental retardation. Once a child is born with PKU, the couple has a one-in-four chance that they will have another child with the disease. The simplicity of this test, the devastating condition, and the fortunate fact that the disease can be prevented by a strict diet, has made PKU testing in newborns almost universal (even mandatory) in the developed world.

Genetic testing may also mean the microscopic examination of the set of forty-six chromosomes in each cell. Breaks, misplacement, additions, and subtractions of material can be seen. Sometimes those changes are associated with disease. For example, a third copy of chromosome 21 is associated with Down's syndrome, a condition that links mental deficiency with distinctive facial features and often cardiovascular defects. This diagnosis can be made by sampling cells from the fetus. Parents are faced with the decision to bring the child to birth or to abort. These chromosomal defects are rarely inherited from a parent but are genetic in the sense that they are caused by an abnormality in the genetic material. In this case, the extra chromosome 21 is usually the result of an error in the formation of the egg or sperm.

Finally, in the last two decades, diagnoses have been made by DNA analysis. Cells are removed from blood or skin and the portion of the chromosome containing the suspected mutated gene is amplified and sequenced by sophisticated procedures to determine whether a gene mutation is present or not. Presence of a mutation indicates the possibility that the person may be affected by the disease and may pass on that possibility to offspring. The possibilities range from relative certainty in a few serious conditions such as Huntington's chorea, in which the presence of a mutated gene predicts that the disease will occur sometime in the future, to statistically based probabilities for most known genetic conditions. Also, the seriousness of many conditions may vary greatly. For example, the skin disease called neurofibromatosis, which has a genetic cause, can appear mildly as spotty discolorations of the skin (café-au-lait spots) or severely as massive outgrowths of flesh, the condition of the famed Elephant Man.

In the mid-1960s, amniocentesis, in which amniotic fluid is withdrawn by needle from the pregnant uterus for examination of fetal cells, came into use. This made possible prenatal testing, with the option of abortion should the test show a serious fetal defect. The most common of these was Down's syndrome, which occurs about once in every eight hundred births, but more frequently in women over the age of forty. Should the amniocentesis reveal a fetal abnormality, the parents could choose abortion. In the early days of the procedure, some physicians refused to perform it unless the woman agreed to abort an affected fetus. Some denounced this ostensibly beneficial procedure as a "search-and-destroy mission."

In the 1990s, preimplantation genetic diagnosis (PGD), already noted in topic 6, was invented. If one or both spouses are concerned that their offspring might suffer from a genetic defect (probably because one or both carries the gene associated with the defect), they can have an embryo created by in vitro fertilization. Out of the tiny cluster of cells formed when ovum and sperm are fertilized in a dish, one cell is plucked and tested for the suspected genetic defect. If that cell is free of the undesirable mutation, the remaining cells are implanted in the woman's uterus and go on to pregnancy. If the cell is affected, the fertilized ovum is discarded. While this procedure would be equivalent to an immoral abortion for any person who held that human life begins at fertilization, many persons can accept this procedure as an alternative to the abortion of a fetus growing in the womb. Even many persons who are distressed by discarding a very early embryo accept this as the lesser of two evils: life is given to a healthy child rather than an affected one.

Presently PGD is used to test for a small range of serious single-gene defects that can be readily detected by chromosomal analysis. It is expensive and requires that the couple conceive by in vitro fertilization rather than by coital reproduction. PGD can be used to determine gender. When a disease is known to be associated with gender (X linked), parents can choose not to implant the embryo. Yet, in the absence of any concern about disease, it allows parents to select the gender of their future child. Also, parents who hope to engender a child who will be a compatible stem cell transplant donor for a living, sick child have undergone PGD testing. Even wider uses are in the offing: tests for other genetically based diseases such as Alzheimer's disease or cancer. These future applications test for the risk of a disease, not its presence. If the risk actually eventuates in disease, onset will probably occur in the far future with variable seriousness. Also, this procedure could be the vehicle for the so-called designer genes, modified to "enhance" the qualities of the fetus, according to the desires of the parents, once this becomes feasible. Thus, PGD forces us to the edge of eugenics, discussed later in this topic.

The ability to diagnose genetic disease with considerable accuracy offers persons important options: those who are carriers of defective genes can decide not to have children, fetuses with genetic defects can be aborted, women with a high risk of inherited breast cancer can choose a preventive mastectomy, or persons learning that they have a gene mutation inevitably leading to a devastating degenerative disease, such as Huntington's chorea, may commit suicide (although few do). Dr. Wexler, having decided not to learn whether she has the fatal gene, prefers to live with the even odds that she will or will not develop the disease. If she does, she knows she can do nothing since there is no effective treatment. If she were to consider having a child, she would probably make a different decision since any child she might bear could carry the gene.

The medical management of a variety of diseases can be modified and improved when their genetic nature is understood. In the case of Jane K., the gene tests could reveal the presence of mutations in two genes, one on chromosome 17, the other on chromosome 13. (Mutations are more prevalent in Ashkenazi Jews but occur in all ethnic groups so far studied.) Tests are most informative when the family history shows a definite pattern of disease. The tests reveal not the presence of disease but a possibility that disease might appear. Thus, someone who tests positive for the gene mutations may or may not become a cancer patient. Also, since breast cancer has many causes, a negative test does not guarantee freedom from future cancer. In Jane K.'s case , the family history is sketchy. Her physician would not recommend the test without better information. If one relative, for example, her aunt, did have cancer late in life, the test might be offered. If the test were done and proved positive, Jane would face the problem of informing relatives (who may not wish to know) and imposing on them the problem of determining what to do (should preventive mastectomy be chosen?). Also, the testing of unconsenting children and gaining information about a dismal future that might never happen is unadvisable.

All of these techniques reflect the major ethical problem of clinical genetics: what is the right course to take in informing persons about the possible futures revealed by genetic diagnosis, and what is the right course to take for individuals who receive that information? Many ethicists recommend that full information should be given; however, once the news is delivered, fully and honestly (which in most cases means warning the patient that the genetic diagnosis estimates the probability rather than certainty of future disease, as well as its probable seriousness), the patient must decide. Genetic counseling for predictive tests such as these, now a developed art, usually does not go beyond providing accurate information and offering patients choices. Although the geneticist will often recommend how a patient might proceed if a test is positive, for example, advising regular mammograms and providing information about the possibility of a preventive mastectomy, the choice of action is clearly left to the patient. The principle of autonomy, firmly ensconced in clinical medicine, prevails in genetic medicine. Some ethicists disagree with this approach, judging that when genetic testing reveals low probabilities that a fatal condition for which there is no therapy may be in the offing, the test should not be offered the patient (unless, of course, the patient demands it).

Autonomy, however, cannot carry the weight in genetics that it does in clinical medicine. In clinical medicine, patients have the right to decide about treatments that affect their well-being. In genetic medicine, many other persons are involved since the culprit in a genetic disease is a defective gene or chromosome circulating through a kinship. The screening of large populations for certain genetic conditions is a particular problem. Genetic screening does not test for a disease but for the presence of genetic indications of the possibility of disease or the possibility of passing that possibility to offspring. Many groups have a high incidence of certain conditions—Ashkenazi Jewish people have a high risk of Tay-Sachs disease, a progressive neurological degeneration that slowly kills infants; African American people are at high risk of sickle-cell anemia; Greeks carry genetic mutations that contribute to serious blood diseases. However, broad screening tests have undesirable effects as well.

One of those undesirable effects is the stigmatizing of a certain population as bearers of a disease or risk of disease. When the genetics of sickle-cell anemia associated that condition with African Americans, the association, very incorrectly interpreted, reinforced discrimination. Carriers of one copy of the gene were, quite wrongly, described as having the disease. Since sickle-cell disease does cause pathological reactions at high altitudes, African Americans found themselves disadvantaged in obtaining jobs as pilots and flight attendants, and admission to the Air Force Academy was restricted. Beyond these particular discriminations, the relation between genetic disease and race is highly debated. Certainly, patterns of susceptibility to disease vary with broad classifications of the human population, but whether those broad classifications relate to race or to the geographical origins of populations is unclear. It is not at all scientifically clear that racial classifications have any genetic basis. So, the discovery of a new drug that reduces death from heart disease among African Americans or the ability to diagnose breast cancer in women of Ashkenasi Jewish origins are valuable surrogates for the underlying genetics of heart disease and breast cancer but do not mark this or that definable population as bearers of a racially characteristic gene. The claim that race is genetically defined opens the debate into eugenics, as we will see in the next section.

It is certainly laudable to detect disease or potential disease, but is it equally laudable to eliminate the disease by eliminating its victim, to mark the surviving victim as defective, or to stigmatize a group as carriers of a defect? Should information be gathered that can be used by others, such as employers, insurers, and government, to the detriment of the persons tested? Should a diagnosis be offered when there is no treatment for the disease? Should information be provided that is extremely difficult to interpret without adequate consoling and education?

The U.S. President's Commission for the Study of Ethical Problems in Medicine endorsed programs for genetic screening, counseling, and education "when they are established with concrete goals and specific procedural guidelines founded on sound ethical and legal principles." Those principles are preservation of confidentiality, respect for personal autonomy, improved knowledge about genetics, provision of benefit, and equity in access. The essential message of the report is that genetic screening should serve the decisions and welfare of individuals and that "the goals of a 'healthy gene pool' or a reduction in health costs cannot justify compulsory genetic screening." Other bioethical advisory bodies around the world have reached similar conclusions.[2] This wise advice draws genetic medicine out from under the dark cloud of eugenics. But not quite.

GENETICS AND EUGENICS

A journalist interviewed Sir (Dr.) Thomas Shakespeare, a British scientist. Dr. Shakespeare, who prefers "Tom" to either of his prestigious titles (he cannot escape his prestigious name), is an achondroplastic dwarf. He and many of his family inherited a defect in a gene that relates to the growth of bones. Tom and the journalist discussed what the journalist described as "one of the most profound and layered questions raised by recent genetics. . . . Do we as a species still want babies born with genetic disabilities?" Science is revealing the genetic basis for genetic ailments, counted now at around seven thousand. It can diagnose many of these disorders in the womb. It is moving toward treatments that might correct them in their earliest stages. The journalist admired these advances but worried that "it is difficult to draw a line where we stop improving our species." Tom responded, "People ask me all the time, 'Wouldn't you rather have been not short?' But that's almost like saying, 'Wouldn't you rather have not been born?'" The journalist opined, "The problem is that it may eventually become possible not just to cull embryos associated with dwarfism, but also to screen out baldness, pug noses or homosexuality, or even to choose the embryo most likely to get into Yale."[3]

The title of that newspaper column about Dr. Shakespeare was "The New Eugenics." This title expresses a deep concern associated with the incredible growth of genetic science. The "new" eugenics differs from the "old" eugenics because today there is a genetic science that has, in the past fifty years, revealed the biochemical and biophysical structures that generate the shape, the organs, and the functions of living beings, from bacteria to humans. The old eugenics lacked that scientific base. Indeed, the name "eugenics" does not itself refer to a science; rather, it is a philosophy that entails speculation about which humans are to be valued over others. This speculation goes far back: Plato's *Republic* suggests practices of human breeding that would produce the "best and bravest" citizens. Plato reminds his hearers that they breed dogs and horses to get the best stock and asks why they should not mate the best men and women to get the best children and prevent the inferior from breeding (*Republic* V, 459–62).

In the nineteenth century, Plato's ideas won a champion, Francis Galton, who coined the word "eugenics" (Greek for "good breeding") for the thesis that the human race might be improved by deliberately multiplying desirable human qualities and eliminating undesirable ones through selective breeding. His ideas quickly spread in intellectual circles in Great Britain and, in particular, in America, where educated citizens worried that their white, Anglo-Saxon, Protestant nation was doomed to degeneration from the vast immigration of people from cultures considered inferior. They were distressed at the numbers of "feebleminded persons," a label that covered not only persons suspected of mental defects but the uneducated, unemployed, and, in their eyes, immoral denizens of immigrant ghettos (and sometimes even of the rural, "hillbilly" country). Many leading Americans, including President Theodore Roosevelt, promoted the eugenics movement.

The eugenics movement had as its only scientific tool observation of physical and behavioral characteristics that seemed to run in families. Eugenicists endlessly collected and counted traits as different as height and hair color, diligence, shiftlessness, leadership, and criminality. They intensively studied richly endowed families and, more frequently, degenerate clans, where ignorance and violence reigned. They endorsed "positive" eugenics, the deliberate selection of desirable physical and behavioral traits through reproductive choices (desirable traits, of course, were those of the educated, white, Protestant American). However, "negative" eugenics was an inevitable implication: was it possible to "breed out" undesirable characteristics by preventing reproduction, either voluntarily or involuntarily. Eugenicists frequently asserted that support of these defectives burdened the taxpaying community. Even worse, these feebleminded people were propagating their unfit kind. It seemed only reasonable to prevent them by sterilization from passing on their feeblemindedness.

At the beginning of the twentieth century, a number of American states required sterilization of the feebleminded released from prisons and asylums (considered a progressive law). Three decades later, the Nazi's eugenics policies burgeoned into a diabolic plan to eliminate wholesale the Jewish inhabitants of Europe, as well as other "inferior" groups, such as Gypsies, and "defectives," such as homosexuals. In the three years following the promulgation of the German Eugenic Sterilization Law of 1933, 225,000 people were sterilized under orders from the hereditary health courts. The eugenics program turned explicitly anti-Semitic with the Nuremberg Laws of 1935, which prohibited marriage between persons of different racial backgrounds, and in 1939, the sterilization program was supplemented with a euthanasia program to eliminate from society the burden of "useless eaters."

While the political uses of eugenics wreaked their havoc (without noticeably "improving" the human race), the rapidly evolving science of genetics was revealing what shoddy, sham science the eugenicists employed. In 1935, a prominent genetic scientist wrote that "eugenics is a hopelessly perverted movement . . . powerless to work any change for the good and [doing] incalculable harm by lending scientific basis to advocates of race and class prejudice."[4] Still, this scientist and many others proficient in the new scientific field of genetics hoped that they could find ways to bend their science to the abolition of disease and to the enhancement of human powers. Eugenics was gone, but genetic engineering and genetic enhancement were increasingly extending human powers over the human heritage.

Ethicists did not remain on the sidelines. Theologian Joseph Fletcher announced himself an enthusiastic supporter of eugenic sterilization. Voluntary sterilization is an act of rational freedom, and compulsory sterilization is a matter of social justice: "It is impossible to see," he wrote, "how the principle of social justice . . . can be satisfied if the community may not defend itself and is forced to permit the continued procreation of feeble-minded or hereditarily diseased children."[5] Fletcher praised the potential of genetic and reproductive science. "It seems to me that laboratory reproduction is radically human compared to conception by ordinary heterosexual intercourse. It is willed, chosen, purposed, and controlled and surely these are among the traits that distinguish *Homo sapiens*. . . . I cannot see how humanity or morality are served by genetic roulette sexually."[6] "Genetics is the real frontier," he exclaimed, "revealing exciting possibilities of quality control for our children."[7] In Fletcher's view, control was the very essence of rationality.

To its critics, the new genetics implied increased power to abuse and exploit. Theologian Paul Ramsey vigorously disputed Fletcher and pugnaciously opposed the new genetics. As a Christian theologian, he asserted the biblical view that man is a being whose dignity does not consist in assuring that those who come after us will be better than we. The Christian does not see any "absolutely imperative end of genetic control or improvement." While Ramsey did advocate "an ethics of genetic duty" in which Christians would adopt policies of restricted reproduction, by voluntary abstinence, for the sake of future generations, he seriously doubted the capability of any human to select the "ideal" genotypes for eugenic purposes. He judged the screening of the unborn or newly born to be a species of "statistical morality, cost-effectiveness analysis and . . . an ethics of the 'greatest net benefit' . . . [leading to] the vanishing of the individual into the mass."[8] Genetic control must respect values other than improved health. Among these, Ramsey chose to dwell on the value of maintaining the unitive and procreative purposes of sex and marriage. Ethicist Dan Callahan was equally concerned that the eagerness to eliminate genetic disease could diminish respect for those who suffer from it. "How can we both manage to live humanely with genetic disease and yet to conquer it at the same time?" he asked.[9]

The new genetics does provide the scientific tools for a new eugenics. Should the shadow of an immoral eugenics inhibit progress in discovering further tools toward genuine improvement in the human condition? The debate over genetic engineering probes that question.

GENETIC ENGINEERING

The term *genetic engineering* is terribly vague and, to the casual ear, sounds pejorative, even sinister. However, it refers to the remarkable discovery during the 1980s of a variety of techniques to modify bits and pieces of the genome. Mutations can be forced on a section of chromosome in a test tube, changing the expression of proteins. If the function of the proteins is known, we can make them stronger or eliminate them for various purposes. Most remarkably, *recombination* allows scientists to splice DNA from another part of the genome or from another genome into the chromosome. The gene that produces human insulin, for example, can be inserted into the genome of a bacterium, causing the bacterium to make human insulin. This engineering has become a standard tool of molecular genetics, applicable in plants, animals, and humans. But its sinister tone, echoing some genuine ethical problems, arouses anxiety.

In 1980, the leaders of Protestant, Catholic, and Jewish faiths in the United States signed a letter to President Jimmy Carter. The letter began,

> We are rapidly moving into a new era of fundamental danger, triggered by the rapid growth of genetic engineering. Albeit, there may be opportunity for doing good; the very term suggests the danger. Who shall determine how human good is best served when new life forms are being engineered? Who shall control genetic experimentation and its results which could have untold implications for human survival? Who will benefit and who will bear any adverse consequences, directly or indirectly? These are not ordinary questions. These are moral, ethical, and religious questions. They deal with the fundamental nature of human life and the dignity and worth of the individual human being.

The religious leaders exclaimed, "Those who would play God will be tempted as never before."[10]

President Carter forwarded the letter to his Commission for the Study of Ethical Problems in Medicine. The commission responded in *Splicing Life: The Social and Ethical Issues of Genetic Engineering with Human Beings.* This report addresses the question of how far we should go toward changing nature, mixing species, controlling evolution, or, in the words of the religious leaders, "playing God."

The report noted that deliberate modification of life forms has long been a human preoccupation (remember Plato's remarks), warned about embarking on genetic adventures that might perpetuate serious mistakes in all species, speculated on the evolutionary effects of genetic engineering, and cautioned about the risks of making changes when so much uncertainty about the function of genes remains. The commission noted that, when it inquired from the religious leaders about the meaning of the metaphor "playing God," the scholars of all faiths represented interpreted it in a positive way. They found in their scriptures no prohibition against changing nature and, indeed,

Catholics, Protestants, and Jews maintain that humans are invited to partici- pate in the divine work of creation as "cocreators."

In 1965, the technical possibilities for such godlike intervention were still remote. They quickly moved from the laboratory to the clinic. *Gene ther- apy*, the repair of gene mutations that cause disease, was the first target. The seminal idea is to extract a functioning gene, insert it into a vector, usually a virus, and send it into the chromosomes of the affected person (sometimes in a culture outside the body, sometimes by directly inserting it into the organ of interest, such as the liver), where it will replace the mutated gene. This semi- nal idea has been extremely difficult to translate into physical reality. It has proven nearly impossible to target precisely the part of the body where the gene expresses itself. Several hundred experiments have been tried, with little success and with some tragedies, such as the death of Jesse Gelsinger.

This form of gene therapy is called *somatic* since it targets the body cells where the deficient production of some enzymes causes disease. Another form of gene therapy is more dramatic. It aims to knock out the diseased gene not in the body cells of the sick person but in his or her *germ cells*, the repro- ductive cells of the gonads. If this were accomplished, the disease would not be passed on to any children of the affected person. This technique could po- tentially wipe inherited disease from the face of the earth. It would be the ul- timate conquest of disease. However, the strongest ethical objections have been raised against germ cell treatment. These objections arise from the pro- found uncertainty associated with changing the human genome. The poten- tial for mistakes is high, and in germ cell treatment, those mistakes would be multiplied through generations. Most bioethicists reject germ cell treatment "until it is proven safe," then wonder how it would be possible to make such a proof.

The ultimate feat of genetic engineering would be the extension of the human lifespan. We no longer search for a fountain of youth; we hunt for genes that propel living things toward death. This is a treasure hunt, for not only are the findings exciting and valuable; they also are hidden everywhere in life, both within the organism and in its environment. Years ago, scientists learned that mice on a rigorous diet lived 40 percent longer than their fatter mates. Of course, some biological mechanism, rooted in genes, must lie be- hind this fact, and gradually, many treasures hidden in many places have been found. One of the most fascinating was the discovery that the end of every chromosome is capped with a *telomere*, like the plastic end of a shoelace. Each time a cell divides, the telomeres of its chromosomes are slightly reduced; fi- nally, the cell dies (the demise of a cell has the wonderful scientific name *apoptosis*). The replication of telomeres is directed by an enzyme, telomerase, and the gene that turns on and off telomerase has been identified on chromosome 14. If telomerase is added to cells, they live through many more divisions than they would otherwise. Is the telomerase gene, TPE1, the secret of longevity? Could manipulation of the enzymes it produces extend life? Could drugs be made to mimic its work?

The answer to aging is far more complex. It would be wrong to think that the telomerase gene is the "longevity gene" or even that there is a longevity gene. Many other genes that control many other aspects of the phenomenon of aging have been identified (some scientists estimate that almost half of the human genome contributes in some way to aging). Some speed up or slow down growth and change metabolism; others clean up cell products that are destructive; still others block chemical messages implicated in diseases like cancer or heart disease. It is far from clear how each of these genes functions and even less clear how they all collaborate. Some of these genes have been found only in insects; a few have been discovered in humans. The hunt is under way but has a long way to go.

The bioethical question is obvious: is it a good thing to extend human life? The obvious answer is, of course, that's what we try to do by eating good food, maintaining good habits, and getting good health care! But the problems, too, are obvious. We certainly do not wish to extend our natural four score and ten to five score and ten if that last score (i.e., twenty years) is filled with all the ills that flesh is heir to. We must not only retard dying; we must eliminate the defects of aging as well. Also, social problems must be expected. Demography already demonstrates that longer-living populations create imbalances in cultural, economic, and environmental aspects of social life. If we move from natural forces that extend life to scientifically enhanced longevity, many questions call for serious consideration: can a society's resources sustain more people, more people of a certain age, more sick people who need health care, or more healthy people who want jobs or social security?

Many, perhaps most, people desire to live long. The principle of autonomy would endorse that desire and support efforts to find ways to retard senescence and death. The principle of beneficence would ask how and why extended life is a benefit and whether it would be a benefit if accompanied by the debility of aging. The principle of justice must ask how success in this venture would shift the burdens and benefits in communities? Would the prolongation of life come only to the privileged? What costs would years of extended life impose on the younger generations or on the environment? Bioethics has a whole agenda of issues surrounding this ultimate genetic engineering. We will say more about this in topic 10 on neuroscience when we discuss enhancement.

BEHAVIORAL GENETICS

People have always known that physical features, such as hair and eye color, height and weight, large noses and protruding chins, run in families. Characteristics other than physical ones seem to be passed through families: musical talent, executive ability, scholarship, piety, competitiveness, aggressiveness. The eugenics movement was much more interested in behavioral than in physical inheritance. Its proponents were eager to prove that ignorance, poverty, and criminality were inherited, were racially endemic and could not be eradicated by education or improved conditions. Properly scientific geneticists ignored the eugenicists' claims and focused on finding the genetic origins of physical traits, particularly the physical manifestations of genetic disease. Now, with our wealth of genetic information, attention returns to behavioral genetics in a much more scientific fashion than in the old eugenics.

Sociological and psychological studies have long attempted to sort out how much human behavior is shaped by nature, that is, by its evolution and genetics, or by nurture, that is, by rearing, education, and social environment. Today, the polarities of nature and nurture are considered overly simplified: a complex interaction of multiple factors goes into the making of behavior. Still, the association between the DNA in our chromosomes and our ways of acting in the world is endlessly fascinating. Do violence, homosexuality, or artistic creativity come from a gene? Although intriguing data suggests some correlation between specific genes and certain behavior traits, few definitive answers are, as yet, forthcoming.

Still, those tentative correlations are quickly transformed into certitudes in the media. A British report on behavioral genetics provides an example: this carefully nuanced document stated that despite a wealth of scientific detail about behavioral genetics, it is misleading to say that there is "a gene for behavior X" or to imply that genes determine behavior or that genetic information as such does not absolve persons from responsibility. The report then cautiously suggested that a judge might be justified in considering genetic information about criminality, along with environmental or psychological information, when issuing a sentence in a criminal case. This cautious opinion made a bold headline in the *London Times*: "Criminal Gene 'Should Mean Lighter Sentence.'"[11]

Such simplification and sensationalism anticipates the future ethical problems with behavioral genetics. If, as many geneticists believe, almost all human behavior derives from a multiplicity of genes interacting with a complex biological and social environment, any simple genetic explanation of behavior will be misleading. Yet, many parties who are intensely interested in human behavior, from educators to judges, from generals to wardens, from ideologues to bigots, may seize on fragmentary information to classify, disqualify, or incarcerate. If, on the other hand, a solid demonstration of genetic causality for some behavior emerges, major social institutions, from schools to courts to legislatures, may have to be reformulated. Our social institutions and our explanations of behavior are permeated with a belief in voluntary, intelligent sources of choice and behavior. These beliefs are challenged by genetic determinism. We shall say more about determinism in topic 10 on neuroscience.

Scientific genetics has generated extraordinary results. The genetic basis for many diseases is better understood. Although very few genetic cures have emerged, diagnostic procedures like that considered by Jane K. are appearing rapidly. All of the people of Iceland are now research subjects: the extraordinary homogeneity of that population prompted a commercial research firm, Decode Genetics, to approach the government and obtain permission to use the health records of the entire nation and to invite citizens to collaborate in studies. The first fruits of this unique study are appearing: genes associated with osteoporosis and cardiovascular disease have been identified. Diagnostic tests will soon be available. These advances, unquestionably positive, raise questions: do people want to know that they live at increased risk of osteoporosis or Alzheimer's disease? What should they do if no prevention or cure is available? Will the information affect their insurance status, their work activities, their reproductive plans? Should the people of Iceland serve as a nation of guinea pigs, signed up by their government as a pool of genetic information?

Bioethics came into being as the eugenics debates were waning and as the debates over the new molecular genetics and its personal and social implications were beginning. From concerns over screening and fears about genetic engineering, the most fundamental questions of human morality have been raised and the old eugenics haunts the new genetics in more scientific guises. In the era of bioethics, those debates have been, in the words of one scientist, "posed with more precision . . . [and] abstract questions about right and wrong [have been reduced] to a series of rather clearly defined situations in which decisions must be reached in relatively concrete terms."[12] The result of those debates has been the adoption of policies and programs in genetic research and in genetic medicine that aim to cure disease, respect the autonomy of individuals, and repudiate utilitarian and eugenic perspectives. At the same time, new questions appear with each new technical innovation.

NOTES

1. D. Suzuki and P. Knudtson, *Genethics: The Clash between the New Genetics and Human Values* (Cambridge, MA: Harvard University Press, 1989).

2. President's Commission on Ethical Problems in Medicine, "Screening and Counseling for Genetic Conditions" (1993), in *Source Book in Bioethics*, ed. A. Jonsen, R. Veatch, and L. Walters (Washington, DC: Georgetown University Press, 1998); Nuffield Council on Bioethics, *Genetic Screening*, 1993; *Mental Disorders and Genetics. The Ethical Context*, 1998; *Genetics and Human Behavior*, 2002.

3. N. Kristof, "The New Eugenics," *New York Times*, July 4, 2003, A21.

4. H. Muller, *Out of the Night: A Biologist's View of the Future* (New York: Vanguard Press, 1935), ix.

5. Joseph Fletcher, *Morals and Medicine* (Princeton, NJ: Princeton University Press, 1954), 168.

6. Fletcher, *Morals and Medicine*, 168.

7. Joseph Fletcher, *Humanhood: Essays in Biomedical Ethics* (Buffalo, NY: Prometheus Press, 1979), 88.

8. P. Ramsey, *Fabricated Man: The Ethics of Genetic Control* (New Haven, CT: Yale University Press, 1970), 7, 31.

9. D. Callahan, "The Meaning and Significance of Genetic Disease," *Ethical Issues in Human Genetics*, ed. B. Hilton (New York: Plenum Press, 1973), 89.

10. President's Commission for the Study of Ethical Problems in Medicine, "Splicing Life: The Social and Ethical Issues of Genetic Engineering, Appendix B," in *Source Book in Bioethics*, ed. A. Jonsen, R. Veatch, and L. Walters, 219–313.

11. T. Lezemore, "Genes, Behavior and the Media," *Hastings Center Report* (November–December 2002): 6; Nuffield Council on Bioethics, *Genetics and Human Behavior*, 2002.

12. R. Morison, quoted in A. Jonsen, *The Birth of Bioethics* (New York: Oxford University Press, 1998), 178.

BIBLIOGRAPHY

Boylan, M., and K. Brown. 2002. *Genetic Engineering*. Upper Saddle River, NJ: Prentice Hall.

Buchanan, A., D. Brock, and N. Daniels. 2000. *From Chance to Choice: Genetic Justice*. New York: Cambridge University Press.

Carson, R., and M. Rothstein, eds. 2002. *Behavioral Genetics*. Baltimore: Johns Hopkins University Press.

Chapman, A., and M. Frankel. 2003. *Designing Our Descendants: The Promises and Perils of Genetic Modification*. Baltimore: Johns Hopkins University Press.

Guttman, D., A. Griffiths, D. Suzuki, and T. Cullis. 2002. *Genetics: A Beginner's Guide*. Oxford: Oneworld Publications.

Kevles, D. 1985. *In the Name of Eugenics*. Cambridge, MA: Harvard University Press.

Mahowald, M. 2000. *Genes, Women, and Equality*. New York: Oxford University Press.

Mehlman, M., and J. Botkin. 1998. *Access to the Genome: The Challenge to Equality*. Washington, DC: Georgetown University Press.

Nuffield Council on Bioethics. 1993. *Genetic Screening: Ethical Issues, Mental Disorders and Genetics*. London.

Nuffield Council on Bioethics. 2002. *Genetics and Human Behavior: The Ethical Context*. London.

Parens, E., and A. Asch, eds. 2000. *Prenatal Testing and Disability Rights*. Washington, DC: Georgetown University Press.

President's Commission on Ethical Problems in Medicine. 1998 [1993]. "Screening and Counseling for Genetic Conditions." In *Source Book in Bioethics*, ed. A. Jonsen, R. Veatch, and L. Walters. Washington, DC: Georgetown University Press.

President's Commission on Ethical Problems in Medicine. 1998 [1982]. "Splicing Life: The Social and Ethical Issues of Genetic Engineering with Human Beings." In *Source Book in Bioethics*, ed. A. Jonsen, R. Veatch, and L. Walters. Washington, DC: Georgetown University Press.

Reich, W., ed. 1995. "Eugenics," "Gene Therapy," "Genetic Counseling," "Genetic Engineering," "Genetic Testing and Screening," "Genetics and Human Behavior," and "Genome Mapping and Sequencing," *Encyclopedia of Bioethics*. New York: Macmillan.

Suzuki, D., and P. Knudtson. 1989. *Genethics: The Clash between the New Genetics and Human Values*. Cambridge, MA: Harvard University Press.

Walters, L., and J. Palmer. 1997. *The Ethics of Human Gene Therapy*. New York: Oxford University Press.

Watson, J. 2003. *DNA: The Secret of Life*. New York: Random House.

• *Topic 10* •

Neuroscience

"New Brain Scans Read the Mind"

A Democratic voter was having his head examined. He lay inside a magnetic resonance imaging (MRI) scanner, while neuroscientists viewed a screen that showed parts of his brain lighting up as he watched a series of political commercials. The scientists noted that a picture of the Democratic candidate activated the reflexive area of the brain, the ventromedial prefrontal cortex; when the Republican candidate appeared, the cognitive area, the dorsolateral prefrontal cortex, lighted up. One scientist said of the study's subjects, "It seems as if they are really identifying with their own candidate, whereas when they see the opponent, they use their rational apparatus to argue against him." When shown a Republican ad featuring the September 11, 2001, terrorist attacks, Democrats also showed more activity in the amygdala, the part of the brain that responds to danger, than did Republicans. Presumably, said the scientists, Democrats considered recall of that event an advantage to the Republican candidate, hence, a threat. Another researcher theorized that Democrats are generally more alarmed by any use of force than Republicans are. The research and the interpretations go on.[1]

Two rhesus monkeys in a university laboratory guide the cursor on a computer screen just by thinking about it. The cursor controls the reaching and grasping activities of a robot that rewards the monkey with a drink of fruit juice. The monkeys had first been trained to control the cursor with their hands. Then, after they were accustomed to the game, the cursor was disconnected. The monkeys soon learned that all they needed to do was think about their reward, and they would win it. Tiny wires inserted into their brains sensed the monkey's thoughts and desires and sent them to the computer,

114

without the monkey physically touching the control. Presumably, paralyzed humans could do just as well, or better, moving computer keys, wheel chairs, and knives and forks by will.[2]

Both of these reports come from neuroscientists. This is a new, rapidly evolving field of science in which anatomy, physiology, chemistry, genetics, neurology, psychology, and psychiatry have united to explore the structure and function of nerve cells, singly and woven into the cables and sheets that carry internal and external information throughout the organism. This new science, in which physical structures and processes are so intertwined with psychological states, touches on human experience at almost every point, from emotion to intellection, from sexual attraction to religious meditation, from personality to culture.

These advances have been propelled by the technique of brain imaging. The functioning human brain, encased in a bony citadel, has resisted invasion until recently. Although the occasional bold explorer probed the living brain during open surgery, only since the development of imaging technology such as positron emission tomography (PET) and MRI, or the more advanced functional MRI (fMRI), have investigators been able to see, in intricate detail and vivid color, the brain at work. These techniques picture the flow of glucose and oxygen as electrical energy is consumed when neurons communicate across brain synapses. The brain sciences can chart the intricate cellular changes that effect and reflect behavior. They can go further to pinpoint where and how thought, affection, and action arise and respond to environment and external stimuli.

The rather silly nineteenth-century science called *phrenology* "mapped" the parts of the brain where certain human behaviors were supposed to sit. Antique shops still display plaster busts with sections marked on the skull: combativeness, amiability, amorousness, mirthfulness. Bumps on the skull over those brain areas supposedly revealed the skull owner's personality. The idea that a single spot in the brain performed a single function persisted until it was possible to visualize dynamic activity. Then, it became obvious that although certain large parts of the brain are dominantly associated with certain sorts of activities, every sensation and action and thought sets off intricate connections across the organ.

As research subjects (some healthy, some with neurological conditions) recline in PET and MRI scanners, they perform various tasks in ingeniously planned investigations. In one classic, simple experiment, subjects were ordered to move a particular finger. When they did, those parts of the brain that recognize the words of the oral command and those that govern physical movement are activated. Then, when subjects are invited to move fingers at will, quite different parts of the brain, those presumably having to do with choice, jump into sight. These technologies have made possible extensive mapping of the enormously complex geography of the human brain, revealing brain activity associated with sensation, movement, memory, emotion, choice, and thought. "Mapping" may not be the right metaphor since these studies reveal a constantly moving flow of energy that represents information. They show not a static geography of the brain but a field of vital tissue that resculpts itself as it responds to experience. It is more like a movie than a map.

Bioethics has not caught up with this rapidly expanding field of study. Although philosophers have reflected on the meaning of mind and consciousness in light of the neurosciences, they rarely engage the ethical implications of the advances in neuroscience. Does getting inside Democratic and Republican heads imply that we might learn not only that their brains respond differently but also how to predict their votes, how to control their votes, or how to change them from one party to another? Does a chip that can send signals from a monkey's brain to a robot hint at the possibility of putting a chip into human brains that will direct people to pull a voting-machine lever as directed? Is this vision silly and far-fetched or prophetic of a possible future in which free will is usurped by deliberate, scientifically designed dominance? Certainly, this is an ethical question if anything is. At a conference to initiate the discourse between neuroscience and bioethics, word-maven William Safire, the conference chairman, called for the creation of a new word, "neuroethics."[3]

One of the few exceptions to this neuroethical silence is a published conversation between a leading French philosopher, Paul Ricoeur, and a prominent French neuroscientist, Jean-Pierre Changeux. The latter says, "The question at issue here is how far the knowledge that we have about our brain gives us a new conception of ourselves, a different representation of our ideas, our thoughts and the dispositions that intervene when we make judgments. . . . I would like to see how far we can succeed in matching up these two discourses about the body [the one involving the body and the brain as objects of knowledge by an external observer, the other of the self resting on a representation that we have of our body] in achieving a synthesis that at first sight may seem impossible." Ricoeur agrees with Changeux's statement of the program, but says, "[A]s a philosopher I profess considerable skepticism with regard to the possibility of constituting an overarching discourse of this sort. . . . In the last analysis, we are dealing with two discourses of the body." Philosopher and neuroscientist recognize the paradox: we experience body and mind each in a unique way; yet, science increasingly tells that they seem to be one.[4]

The discourses of philosophy about ethics and of science about the brain are, as it were, two populated shores of an unexplored continent. On one shore, there are centuries of rich philosophical and theological debates about human identity, choice, virtue, responsibility, and social justice; on the other shore, recent neurobiology has built an impressive world of scientific data and theory. The languages spoken on either shore are quite different; yet, in many respects, they seem to be referring to the same thing, the nature and function of the human being as a neuronal organism and as an agent of behavior. The intervening continent that links those two shores is virtually unexplored; neither philosophers nor scientists have seriously attempted to link the two shores in any systematic way. One leading neuroscientist has commented that "we don't even know the right words to carry on this conversation."

Can the terrain of the unknown continent linking ethics and science be opened to exploration? At what points do philosophical discourse about questions of ethics seem to point toward or touch on scientific discourse about neuronal correlates of language, valuing, choosing, emoting, and so forth? How should those points of virtual contact be defined? Does knowing that a part of the brain called the amygdala lights up in sexy situations explain, as the title of a recent book puts it, why we love? Does knowing that sections of the temporal lobe are associated with feelings of spiritual transcendence explain religious belief? Can traditional ways of posing philosophical questions about free will be reconciled with scientific explanations of choosing behaviors? Of what relevance is the evidence about brain pathology to our understanding of moral and criminal accountability? As Changeux says, "Can neuronal man be a moral subject? I have not ceased to reflect on this question, to make a serious attempt to give new meaning to an ethics of the good life—a joyful, humanist ethics compatible with the free exercise of reason." Are these words, uttered by a neurobiologist, the preface to a program of discourse between the two disciplines?

A story frequently cited in neuroscience literature provides a striking example of the way in which the physical brain and psychic life are associated. In 1861, a derelict man, Phineas Gage, died in San Francisco. Thirteen years before, Gage had been the victim of a freak accident. An iron bar had blasted into his left cheek, through the ventromedial region of his frontal lobe and out the top of his skull. Gage lived, his physical capacities intact and his cognitive facilities unimpaired, with one gaping exception: he became incapable of making moral decisions. Neuroscientist Antonio Damasio opens his book, *Descartes' Error: Emotion, Reason and the Human Brain*, with Gage's history.

> Gage had once known all he needed to know about making choices conducive to his betterment. He had a sense of personal and social responsibility. . . . He was well adapted in terms of social convention and appears to have been ethical in his dealings. After the accident, he no longer showed respect for social convention; ethics . . . were violated, the decisions

he made did not take into account his best interest. . . . There was no evidence of concern about his future, no sign of forethought. . . ." [Damasio poses basic questions about] "Gage's status as a human being. May he be described as having free will? Did he have a sense of right and wrong or was he the victim of his new brain design, such that his decisions were imposed upon him and inevitable? Was he responsible for his acts? . . . Gage had lost something uniquely human, the ability to plan his future as a social being."[5]

Damasio then relates the story of one of his own patients, a promising young man whom he calls Elliot. After extensive brain surgery to remove a tumor, Elliot had become "Gagelike": irresponsible, disorganized, reckless, yet still manifesting intelligence and comprehension. Such patients cannot generate the power to move from understanding a moral situation to making a moral choice. This radical destruction of moral personality is not occasioned by the slide from virtue to vice that traditional moralists abhor; it is rooted in the physical brain, in a distinct area of the prefrontal cortex, and is now explicable in terms of neuropsychology, neuroanatomy, and neuropathology.

After describing Gage's lesion and subsequent behavior, Damasio states a theme for neuroethics: "the fact that acting according to an ethical principle requires the participation of simple circuitry in the brain core does not cheapen the ethical principle. The edifice of ethics does not collapse, morality is not threatened and in a normal individual the will remains the will."[6] This is a bold affirmation. What are we to say about that elemental concept of ethics, free will, in the light of the neurosciences? What do the profound claims of philosophers, theologians, and humanists about human dignity and the assumptions of lawyers and judges about culpability and responsibility mean in the light of comparative and evolutionary neuroscience? How should the ethicist look at daily problems of moral duty and dereliction in the light of the brain sciences?

This topic examines two issues that a future neuroethics might study. One of these, the question of free will and responsibility, arises particularly in the neurosciences. The other, enhancement of human nature, is shared between neuroscience and genetics. Both of these questions, however, call for concepts and forms of reasoning that go beyond those current in standard bioethics.

FREE WILL AND RESPONSIBILITY

Novelist Tom Wolfe warned the 2002 commencement audience at Duke University about "the tremendous influence of neuroscience." "If I may reduce with terrible reductiveness, the bottom line of the neurosciences is . . . [that] we are all concatenations of molecules containing DNA, hard wired into a chemical analog computer known as the human brain . . . and your idea that you have a soul or even a self, much less free will, is just an illusion." All the complicated motives of Wolfe's fictional characters and all the aspirations of the graduates for the lives they will make for themselves are but fictions of a "fate preordained."[7] Wolfe has apparently been reading the media stories that chronicle the extraordinary findings of neuroscientists. Now that brain imaging reveals real-time pictures of the brain responding to stimuli and forming electrochemical patterns that correspond to experience, emotion, and intellection, much of the mystery of our lives seems reducible, "with terrible reductiveness," to that capsule of cells, neurons, and chemicals called the brain.

Wolfe's commencement proclamation about determinism poses a fundamental question about the implications of the neurosciences. Wolfe is, of course, not the first to proclaim "fate preordained." Long before the neurosciences, philosophers such as the Epicureans and theologians like John Calvin were convinced that free will was but an illusion. These savants could not see the vivid images of neural activity; nor could they cite elaborate scientific data to support their speculative claims. Yet, they, like Wolfe and others who read of these discoveries, clearly saw that if choice and thought are only the work of the "hard wiring in a chemical analog computer," the claims we make about responsibility, freedom, moral obligation, and religious belief are not what they seem. Do the theories and data of the neurosciences inevitably lead to such firm declarations of determinism? Does modern neuroscience negate common understanding of free will and erase our vaunted sense of human uniqueness?

Free will is not free wheeling, that is, choice rolling along without brake or impulse. Almost all philosophers acknowledge that choice is caused by prior events and influences. Nevertheless, free choice, in some special way, seems to come from ourselves; we seem to be in control. Aristotle wrote that "a voluntary act would seem to be one of which the originating cause lies in the agent himself, who knows the particular circumstances of his action."[8] What might this originating cause be? Is it some spirit floating above brain and body? Or is it somehow embedded within the brain, body, and physical world but in a way quite different from the cause-and-effect relationships we find in nature? Is it nothing but an illusion? Since the debut of philosophy, these questions have been asked. We know what no ancient thinker knew, namely, that learning right from wrong—acquiring a conscience—is dependent on neural tissue in the ventromedial prefrontal cortex and on circuitry in the hypothalamus, the amygdala, and cingulate cortices. Damage in that region extinguishes or diminishes the behavior we associate with free, voluntary choice; drugs and devices, such as microchips, seem to affect these behaviors. What would philosophers, familiar with these facts, say about free choice?

There is a temptation to collapse the experience of a range of moral behaviors, such as attributing responsibility, blaming, praising, making excuses, evaluating options, and educating for moral behavior, into assertions about data and theory from empirical science. This is called *reductionism*, and Wolfe admits that he is committing it. Such a statement is easy to make but hard to prove since the evidence is never sufficient. It is, in essence, a large, unprovable metaphysical assertion. *Partial reductionionism* is a more intellectually respectable position. It sees connections and correlations in particular situations, which strongly suggest that the "originating cause" does not "lie within the agent himself." Certain acts in certain circumstances or certain processes under certain conditions can be plausibly demonstrated to be determined, that is, linked in a causal chain in which each link is necessary and sufficient. When we become aware of such links, we might allow for excuses; we might mitigate blame, educate, and admonish rather than punish, forgive, and forget.

Attributing free will is, as one philosopher says, the default position. In the absence of excusing conditions, we assume free and voluntary choice. Excusing conditions, such as loss of muscular control, coercion by threats, psychological and physical abnormalities, all of which we may better understand through the neurosciences, may render the otherwise free individual incapable of choice.[9] On the positive side, the multiple activities that swirl around the choices we describe as free, such as reflection, inquiry, motivation, intention, evaluation, commitment, conversion, regret, criticism, questioning, doubt, and change of mind, suggest that even partial reductionism should be affirmed cautiously. Of course, in principle we will find neurological correlates of each of these activities, but the fact that they flow so copiously around our choices imparts something of a mystery.

Bioethicists constantly refer to the principle of autonomy, as we saw in Part II. When they work in neuroethics, they must plunge into the meaning of autonomy, revisiting the time-honored philosophical debates about free will in light of science. It is their task to redescribe these problems in ways that, as medieval philosophers used to say, "save the appearances," not denying the experience but explaining it so as to complement the scientific data. The paradoxes of free will have never abolished the insistent human need to assign responsibility for actions: praise and blame, reward and punishment are universal human behaviors. These behaviors are, of course, the subject matter of ethics. So, neuroethics must accommodate these activities. What can be made of the daily problems of moral duty and dereliction in the light of the brain sciences? One author, writing about Phineas Gage, asks,

[I]f self-determination lies in a specific bit of tissue, it follows that those who appear not to have it may simply be unlucky: victims of a sluggish brain module. So is it reasonable to blame the Phineas Gages of today for their ways? Should we be unsympathetic to addicts who fail to conquer their habit or punish recidivist criminals?[10]

The assertion that "self-determination lies in a specific bit of tissue" needs the most careful examination. Is the behavior we describe as self-determination in the tissue? Does the tissue cause self-determining acts? Is the bit of tissue a necessary and sufficient cause of behavior? Does the tissue perform certain cellular and neurochemical functions when a person performs a self-determining act? What, indeed, is a self-determining act? An act without any influences other than the mysterious will? These are questions for the complementary dialog between philosophers and neuroscientists.

The neuroscientists will contribute new data and interpretations of neurological physiology and activity to the dialog. They can propose, for example, that persons have dispositions to act in certain ways because neural tracks and pathways are built by every experience and every choice. The brain approaches new situations with multiplex circuitry in place. However, the new experience also reforms that circuitry and does so by processing new information, interpretation, and imagination. The philosophers must take these explanations of the data and explain what choice, freedom, and responsibility might mean in light of them.

The questions and answers of this dialog will inform the policy and practices of major institutions, such as the criminal justice system, the mental-health system, and the educational system. These questions will be unremitting and the answers never definitive. Yet they generate new information, foster new insights, and promote a prudent skepticism about received solutions. We must be wary of unsupported proclamations either of determinism or of freedom. It is intriguing to recall that religion, in Western and Eastern cultures, has often subordinated free will to the omnipotence of God or nature, yet sustained a strong sense of personal responsibility for behavior and for salvation.

Although many philosophers have claimed that the problem of free will and determinism is a "pseudoproblem" because it has no solution, some moral philosophers with a practical bent have not been disconcerted. Aristotle proposes no clear thesis about free will but uses the notion of uncoerced choice to open many crucial questions about moral education. William James, a philosopher deeply immersed in empirical psychology, did not believe that the "free will problem" could be solved in any theoretical or metaphysical way but insisted that, without an affirmation of free will, vast tracts of our moral life make no sense, that moral education and social ethics are useless enterprises, and that free will, expressed in the conviction that our decision "in soul trying moments . . . gives palpitating reality to our moral life and makes it tingle."[11] A practicing bioethicist may not know for certain whether self-determination lies in a specific bit of tissue but must certainly know that praising and blaming, punishment and reward are practices inherent to the moral life and must be conducted intelligently and responsibly.

Attribution of moral responsibility for one's actions is the most urgent question for the practicing bioethicists. Is this person—someone consenting to a medical procedure, deciding to forgo life support, declining genetic information, or, in another area of ethics, accused of a crime—responsible?

William Winslade, a bioethicist, psychotherapist, and lawyer, tells the story of John, a promising young man rising in his occupation. After a serious car accident, he spent nine months in the hospital. He left the hospital a "fulminating paranoid" and came to believe that his mother, with whom he lived, was part of a conspiracy against his life. He shot her dead. Psychiatrists judged him a paranoid schizophrenic, and the judge sent him to a psychiatric hospital where he was confined for twenty-eight years. Winslade evaluated John and found, as did other clinicians, that he showed no signs of mental illness and suggested that John's behavior was due to brain injury sustained at the time of the accident. Winslade suggests that greater attention to diagnosis of brain injury might have suggested a very different approach, namely, treatment instead of confinement. Winslade also refers to a study of fifteen death row inmates showing that all of them had, at some time, suffered traumatic brain injury. This fact was not considered in their defense or sentencing. The fact that brain injury diminishes or destroys the ability to go through the reflective processes associated with free choice does not, in itself, prove that free choice is an illusion or that every person who commits a violent crime is not responsible for that action. It does demonstrate that a scientific and medical knowledge of brain injury may, in specific cases, change the ethical or legal judgment about the case.[12]

ENHANCEMENT OF HUMAN NATURE

Advances in the neurosciences, like advances in genetics, are often prompted by the desire to understand and cure diseases. Current understanding of the neurochemical features of schizophrenia and depression have stimulated the search for an adequate neuropharmacology, drugs that might remedy the devastating effects of these conditions without destroying other aspects of life. Attention deficit hyperactivity disorder (ADHD) is a prominent example. Children who are excessively disruptive in school and at home were once judged as "bad kids." Now brain imaging reveals that many of these children have a neurological dysfunction: those areas of the brain that control impulse and focus attention function at a low level. The drug methylphenidate, or Ritalin, can stimulate those centers, rendering the children more attentive and docile. However, many children are diagnosed with this condition without brain imaging: their behavior alone tags them. In fact, many of them may act as they do for reasons quite other than a hypoactive prefrontal cortex: the social and economic settings in which they live and learn may often be the major contributor to their aberrant behavior. Yet, when the drug "solves" the apparent problem, these other influences are ignored and remain unchanged. Here proper neuroscience must direct appropriate therapy.

The use of pharmaceuticals aimed at correcting a neurologically based problem fits the model of medicine. However, other drugs, developed on the basis of neurological science, can go beyond correction of defects. Many drugs aim to improve performance and appearance, such as drugs for male impotence and baldness. Drugs enhance memory, sharpen perception for tasks like piloting an aircraft, and augment strength in athletics. As scientific understanding proceeds, we shall certainly see drugs that will make thinking faster and clearer. In addition to drugs, other technologies such as chips implanted in the brain to affect certain functions (controlling epileptic seizures, for example, just as a pacemaker controls the heart muscle) are in the offing. The executive monkeys described at the opening of this topic augur what might be done. Indeed, we are seeing the bionic human of fiction becoming reality. One bioethicist commented, "Once you integrate technologies into the brain, you then have to ask yourself, 'is there an end of the non-technological me and the beginning of the technological me, or is it now all me?'"[13]

The distinction between treatment and enhancement is now commonly made in genetics and neurosciences. Some lean on this distinction to mark off the ethically permissible from the impermissible. Yet, it is a distinction without much of a difference. Clearly, the cure of manifest physical and mental deficits and disorders would count as treatment, but where does the spectrum of disease end? Is infertility a disease? Is impotence a disease? Is intellectual "slowness" a disease? Should we call cosmetic surgery treatment or enhancement? Are the "ultimate makeovers" of faces and bodies displayed on television merely the ultimate manifestations of egoism or "cures" for a pathological self-hatred? Human growth hormone (HGH) was originally given to children with a known biochemical deficiency leading to short stature—in this sense, it was clearly treatment. Today, HGH is given to short kids with no evidence of hormonal deficiency—now it is called enhancement. Or is it treatment because it prevents the psychopathology of inadequacy that being short in a tall world reinforces? Also, we continually enhance ourselves and our children by education, physical training, and cultural activities. These enhancements are worthy of praise. Are there enhancements that are acceptable and others that are not?

Those who repudiate enhancement as a legitimate goal suggest that some enhancements violate an order of nature. They complain that we fallible humans lack the wisdom to modify nature for the better. These objections are met by others who ask exactly what lines clearly delimit the "natural" and point out that we fallible humans have been improving the natural condition of life for a millennia. Other objections are more thought provoking. Would access to enhancement technologies widen the rift between the wealthy and the poor? Would enhancements destroy fair competition in employment, athletics, and academia? Would the enhanced acquire power to control the unenhanced? Would new discriminations arise between the enhanced and the unenhanced? Would enhancement be a euphemism for changes that suit the enhanced for tasks and purposes set by their enhancers? Would the ultimate enhancement, the prevention or retardation of aging, fill the world to bursting, imposing an intolerable load on the already burdened environment?

Although mere invocation of the word "enhancement" provides no moral illumination, the problem to which it refers must be taken seriously. Clearly, humans seek, and have always sought, to enhance their lives. Work, building, education, art, and exercise all enhance human life. Socrates might allow us to paraphrase his maxim as "the unenhanced life is not worth living." Clearly also, enhancement can create inequalities, some of which are acceptable, others invidious; enhancement of one characteristic can distort other equally important features of life. There may be some "natural" norm that can help us measure which enhancements are right and which are wrong; yet, philosophers have not agreed on where that natural norm can be found. Bioethicists must deal with every project of enhancement, physical or spiritual, on its own terms. They must ask whether this project injects invidious inequalities into the human community; whether it challenges ethical concepts of fairness and moderation; whether it distracts attention away from equally significant human achievements and values. Aristotle argued that virtue consists in finding a mean between extremes in all human activity and that the mean is discerned by prudent judgment in the circumstances. Bioethicists studying enhancement in genetics and neuroscience might keep this Aristotelian advice in mind.

CONCLUSION

Sir Francis Crick, the codiscoverer of the helical structure of DNA, turned his acute scientific mind to neuroscience. He devoted his last years to proving an "astonishing" hypothesis. He writes, "You, your joys, your sense of personal identity and free will, are in fact no more than the behavior of a vast assembly of nerve cells and their associated molecules. As Lewis Carroll's Alice might have phrased: 'You're nothing but a pack of neurons.' This hypothesis is so alien to the ideas of most people today that it can truly be called astonishing."[14] Crick asserts that a deeper, fuller scientific understanding of how that "pack of neurons" works will satisfactorily explain joy, personal identify, free will, and all else that we attribute to a "self" or, even more mistakenly, to a "soul." The subtitle of Crick's book is "The Scientific Search for the Soul." Of course, he does not expect to find the soul at the end of his search. He fully expects that once enough is known about the pack of neurons, no one will need to wonder where or whether the soul exists. However cogent his scientific explanations might be, does he eliminate the need to make moral judgments about responsibility, freedom, and dignity? Will he admit that his Nobel Prize came to him not because he "deserved" it but because his pack of neurons magnetically attracted it in his direction? Or, in a moment of humility, might he admit that, as Paul Ricoeur told Changeux, "In the last analysis, we are dealing with two discourses of the body."

Neuroethics is a newcomer to bioethics. The neurosciences are themselves newcomers to biological science. They draw together very diverse fields such as psychology and molecular biology. Their investigative methods are constantly evolving. Their explanation of brain activity becomes ever more sophisticated. Bioethics is hardly ready to deal with the neurosciences. It will have to rejoin its intellectual ancestor, moral philosophy, where the questions of human nature and responsibility were pondered. Neuroscience has major implications for major human activities, such as education, marketing, criminal justice, even religion. Its manner of understanding these activities should be complemented by a humanistic appreciation of the human person at their heart.

NOTES

1. "Politics on the Brain," *New York Times*, April 20, 2004, A1, A17.
2. "Monkey Think, Robot Do," *New York Times*, October 13, 2003, A15.

3. W. Safire, "Visions for a New Field of 'Neuroethics,'" in *Neuroethics: Mapping the Field, Conference Proceeding, May 13–14, 2002*, ed. S. Marcus (New York: Dana Press, 2002).

4. P. Ricoeur and J.-P. Changeux, *What Makes Us Think? A Neuroscientist and a Philosopher Argue about Ethics, Human Nature and the Brain*, trans. M. DeBevoise (Princeton, NJ: Princeton University Press, 2000), 27, 29.

5. A. Damasio, *Descartes' Error* (New York: HarperCollins, 1995), 11, 18.

6. Damasio, *Descartes' Error*, xiv.

7. T. Wolfe, "Commencement Speeches," *New York Times*, June 2, 2002, A26.

8. *Nicomachean Ethics* III, iii, 1111a20.

9. K. Shaffner, "Neuroethics: Reductionism, Emergence and Decision-Making Capacities," in Marcus, *Neuroethics*, 30.

10. R. Carter, *Mapping the Mind* (Berkeley: University of California Press, 1989), 27.

11. William James, "The Dilemma of Determinism," in *Writings of William James*, ed. J. J. McDermott (Chicago: University of Chicago Press, 1977), 610.

12. W. Winslade, "Traumatic Brain Injury and Legal Responsibility," in Marcus, *Neuroethics*, 75–81.

13. P. Wolpe, "Neurotechnology, Cyborgs, and the Sense of Self," in Marcus, *Neuroethics*.

14. F. Crick, *The Astonishing Hypothesis: The Scientific Search for the Soul* (New York: Charles Scribner's Sons, 1994).

BIBLIOGRAPHY

Churchland, P. 1994. *The Engine of Reason, The Seat of the Soul: A Philosophical Journey into the Brain*. Cambridge, MA: MIT Press.

Damasio, A. 1994. *Descartes' Error: Emotion, Reason and the Human Brain*. New York: HarperCollins.

Dennett, D. 1984. *Elbow Room: The Varieties of Free Will Worth Having*. Cambridge, MA: MIT Press.

Fisher, H. 2003. *Why We Love: The Nature and Chemistry of Romantic Love*. New York: Henry Holt & Company.

Gazzinga, M. 2005. *The Ethical Brain*. Chicago: University of Chicago Press.

Marcus, S. 2002. *Neuroethics: Mapping the Field*. New York: Dana Press.

Parens, E. 1998. *Enhancing Human Traits: Ethical and Social Implications*. Washington, DC: Georgetown University Press.

President's Council on Bioethics. 2003. *Beyond Therapy: Biotechnology and the Pursuit of Happiness*. Washington, DC: U.S. Government Printing Office, at www.bioethics.gov/reports/beyond therapy.

Winslade, W. 1999. *Confronting Traumatic Brain Injury: Devastation, Hope and Healing*. New Haven, CT: Yale University Press.

Cloning and Stem Cell Research

*I*n 1996, a lamb was conceived and born without any contribution from a ram. The lamb, named Dolly, came into being by cloning: the nucleus of a cell taken from the mammary gland of an adult ewe was inserted into the egg of another ewe that had been emptied of its nucleus. This egg was placed in the womb of a third ewe and carried to term. Thus, Dolly not only had no male parent; she was genetically identical to her mother, who was not the ewe that bore her but the ewe whose mammary cell had started the process.

Soon after Dolly's birth announcement, Raël, prophet of a sect named after him, garbed in white robe and bedecked with gold medallion, appeared at a congressional hearing on cloning. He explained to the astonished senators that in 1972 space aliens told him that they had cloned the human race in their image. They commissioned him to bring to humankind cloning as a scientific technique to breed an improved race destined for eternal life by perpetual repetition of selves (of course, it would be possible to download a person's mind into the cloned body). The members of Congress were not impressed and drafted legislation that forbade human cloning. Soon Raël announced, without providing evidence, that his group had in fact cloned a human baby. The idea of cloning was trumpeted in the media as if it were available at the local supermarket. The recipe sounded easy.

A *clone* is a group of cells or an organism arising asexually from a single ancestral cell, thus genetically identical to it. Farmers and gardeners have cloned plants from ancient times by cutting and planting slips or bulbs. The Greek word *clōn* means a twig or a cutting (a gardener's "slip"). Cloning of animals from germinal cells has become common in animal husbandry, but not until Dolly was an animal cloned from a body (somatic) cell. Once this barrier was crossed, it was clear to scientists that humans could, in principle, be cloned. A living person could, theoretically, have a copy of him- or herself made simply by giving a scientist some cells scraped from his skin. Scientists would extract the nucleus of those cells, containing a complete set of the person's chromosomes, and insert that nucleus into a female egg emptied of its own nucleus, a process called *nuclear transfer* (NT). After an electric shock fused the nucleus and the ovum, the newly made cell would germinate in a dish for a few days, multiplying as if it were an embryo fertilized by sperm. It would then be implanted in the uterus of a willing woman who could bear it to birth. The result would be a genetic copy of the cell donor with the same genetic profile, equivalently an identical twin but of a different generation.

Animals and plants are cloned for economic reasons. It is an efficient way to produce beefier steers or more productive milk cows. Why not clone humans? Cloning might provide a more efficient method of reproduction, which is now, as Joseph Fletcher has called it, a genetic roulette. The Raëlians believe cloning is the equivalent of eternal life, the endless repetition of oneself. A human clone might represent the supreme egoism of its source, who believes he can watch himself grow up again. A child, cloned from cells saved from a dead son or daughter, could give back to bereaved parents a replica of the child they lost. A clone of an ill child is the most compatible organ donor for that child; indeed, a clone could be an organ bank for expected organ failures of its origin. The imagination then takes hold. Clones might be engineered with "designer genes" to make the copies stronger, smarter, more servicable. A football team cloned from the best player in the world would be unbeatable. An army cloned from the bravest of the Green Berets would fight ferociously, and perhaps, the death of its soldiers would be less devastating since they were not strictly anybody's children but only copies. The 1980s film *Boys from Brazil* depicted a cloned pack of Adolf Hitlers. The idea is endlessly intriguing.

The reality is much more complex and much less sensational. A genetic copy is not a human copy. Genes are the codes that direct the building of the chemicals that make up the proteins that make up the body of an organism. Between proteins and personality are a myriad of steps and influences, some of which can be sorted out and others that are bafflingly elusive. Identical twins share the same genome, accounting for their physical similarity, but even that similarity is not exact physical identity. Their psychological and emotional life may be strikingly similar (especially if they are raised in close proximity), but each manifests individual feelings, tastes, and ideas. The many scientific studies that attempt to trace personality and behavioral characteristics to a genetic origin reveal chains of solid causal connections that then tangle and dissipate into wide, hardly traceable webs of connection. It is certain, for example, that a gene called 5-HTT directs the making of a protein that affects the way in which nerve cells react to serotonin, a chemical compound that, among other things, affects mood. It is also clear that many people who have one version of that gene are more susceptible to depression. However, it is "many" people, not all; it is "more susceptible" because depression is also associated with the seriousness and duration of stressful life events. Also, men and women differ in incidence of depression; 5-HTT seems to have nothing to do with this gender difference. This complexity reveals that the path from gene to personality to actual experience is long, winding, and intricate.

Interesting problems of identity and relationship are engendered: Is the cloned person a sibling or a descendant of the donor? Does a shared genome imply a shared identity? Is being a clone any different from being an identical twin? If a project of fashioning clones were devised, would they be cloned for a specific purpose, with characteristics suited to that purpose? Would a clone have to live up to the expectations of its source or its designer? What then would happen to the clone's freedom to develop as an individual? Is copying a genome into another person a sort of identity theft? These questions can be debated endlessly. Despite the fascinating features of cloning, it appears that many persons feel some repugnance at the thought (one bioethicist has called this the "Ugh! factor").

Soon after Dolly's birth, the debates moved into places where policy is made. Congress and Parliament debated and voted on cloning. International organizations issued statements. Bioethics commissions under two American presidents studied the question. In general, human reproductive cloning has not done well in these forums. The influence of religious antipathy toward a process that comes so close to usurping divine creativity has been influential. So radical a departure from the procreative ideal of the family is troubling. Opponents often aver that human cloning is an affront to the dignity of humans: being the mere copy of another person seems demeaning. However, the primary reason that human cloning is so roundly repudiated internationally is the daunting problem of safety. The cloning of animals is not technically easy: many efforts fail and successful clonal implants are often aborted, showing signs of severe anomalies. The prospect of experimental production of human clones almost certainly would produce a similar record. Also, it was suspected that Dolly the clone showed signs of rapid aging: would the clone be born with the physical age of its source? Thus, in the years after Dolly's birth, ethics councils and legislatures around the world condemned cloning as a technique to produce a human child.

STEM CELL RESEARCH

Three years after Dolly's birth, cloning entered the news again in new clothing. Dr. James Thomson of the University of Wisconsin published a paper describing his isolation of *embryonic stem cells* (ESTs) from human embryos left over from assisted reproduction. ESTs are the primitive cells found in the earliest forms of embryos; they are not the cells of any particular tissue, such as bone, brain, or skin, but the forerunners of every kind of cell that the mature organism needs.

During the five days after fertilization, cells divide and shape their two hundred or so cells into a hollow ball, called the *blastocyst*. If fertilization has taken place within a female body, the blastocyst then implants in the wall of the uterus and continues its development into a fetus. If the blastocyst is formed in a laboratory dish, as in in vitro fertilization, it can be transferred to the uterus of a mother or frozen for later transfer.

Alternatively, its development can be stopped by dissecting out the inner mass of some fifty cells. These are the ESTs. At this point they are *pluripotent*, as yet undifferentiated into the some two hundred cell types that make up the living body, among them muscle, skin, nerve, heart, liver, gut, and so forth. In addition to being undifferentiated, they are capable, under proper laboratory conditions, of *proliferating*, that is, continuing to divide in their undifferentiated state. Also, and most important, they can be coaxed by chemical means into becoming a certain cell type, for example, heart cells or nerve cells. In theory, these proliferated and differentiated cells could be transplanted into living bodies, providing *regeneration* for organs and tissues that have been damaged by injury or disease. A new form of medicine, called *regenerative medicine*, exists in the imagination of scientists who anticipate the power of stem cells to make replacements for dead heart muscle, islet cells that no longer make insulin, or the severed cables of glial cells that cannot carry neural messages through the spinal cord. We can watch lab-made movies of mice, whose spinal cords have been severed, recover after a stem cell transplant: from cripples dragging their hind legs, they now scurry again (although rather clumsily).

An elaborate science is developing to describe, explore, and explain this process. That science remains far from complete (if any science can ever be called complete). One of the intriguing questions, for example, is whether *adult stem cells* have properties similar to ESTs. Blood stem cells have long been recognized: they are the primitive cells generated from bone marrow that differentiate into various kind of blood cells, such as red cells that carry oxygen and white cells that fight infection. Other stem cells have been found in mature tissue, such as fat and intestines. These cells appear to have the quality of continued replication, but they do not appear to have pluripotentiality, at least not to the extent possessed by ESTs. Most scientists are interested in understanding more about adult stem cells but at present are skeptical about their contribution to regenerative medicine. Yet, even those scientists who discount the efficacy of adult stem cells concede that scientific study should pursue embryonic and adult forms of stem cells.

Thomson did not clone an embryo to find stem cells. Rather, he took a fertilized human embryo, created by in vitro fertilization, and extracted the inner cell mass where the stem cells are found, thus destroying the embryo. The destruction of a human embryo was the shot that started the stem cell wars. That war was waged in the media, in religious congregations, in scientific associations, and in the legislatures of many nations. However, it is possible to search for stem cells by cloning an embryo by NT. It is this possibility that connected stem cell research with cloning in the public mind, as well as the fact that both techniques of finding stem cells destroy embryos. The second technique was actually realized in 2004, when two Korean scientists announced that they had cloned a human embryo and extracted stem cells from it.

The stem cell war has been fought almost exclusively as a moral dilemma between an absolute right and an absolute wrong. A *New York Times* editorial articulated the dilemma: "Advocates argue that embryonic stem cell research can help cure an array of diseases, including Parkinson's. But abortion opponents say the research destroys embryos and, therefore, violates human life."[1] The public and the political debates have been framed in terms of this stark moral dichotomy. This dichotomy sets up a moral dilemma: advocates and opponents almost universally believe that research leading to improved treatment of serious disease is a good; almost all accept the moral injunction that it is wrong to destroy human life. Thus, the dilemma: choice of one course over the other leads either to violation of a moral injunction or to the repudiation of a human good. We are presented with an either/or moral problem. But let us leave the media and enter the conscience of one who must make decisions about the right course of action.

A scientist (let us call him Damien O') at a British research center has an international reputation for his study of *histocompatibility*, that is, the genetic and biochemical process that enables the tissue of one organism to be transplanted into another organism without rejection. In recent years, he has explored a new direction to understand this process and to seek ways to prevent the disaster of immune rejection of organs, as happened in the tragedy of Jésica Santillán. Scientists like Damien O' realize that stem cells hold the promise of eliminating the problem of immune rejection. It is theoretically possible to take cells from a person whose heart muscle has been destroyed by an infarction and culture that person's own cells into a sheet of heart cells that could replace the damaged segment. In order to obtain stem cells, the recipient of the transplant would be "cloned," that is, one cell of the patient's body, taken from skin, would be inserted into a human ovum donated by a woman; the ovum, properly manipulated, would begin to develop as would a fertilized egg. At about five days of growth, the two-hundred-cell entity would be dissected and the inner cell mass of some fifty cells removed. These would be cultured and then coaxed by chemical manipulation into one cell type, cardiomyocytes, that could be transplanted as new heart muscle. In theory, this transplanted tissue would not be rejected because it was derived from the person's own tissue.

This is the image of regenerative medicine that has captured the public mind: organ transplants will never be rejected again since every patient will get his own regrown organ. This image is, of course, exaggerated. This highly individual therapy, growing a new organ for each patient, would be extremely costly, inefficient, and inequitable. Many scientists even doubt that self-transplants would escape immune rejection. Regenerative medicine will succeed only if another solution for immune rejection can be found. Thus, scientists are exploring the possibility of cell banks or genetic engineering to silence the genes that turn on immune rejection. It is this last technique that fascinates Damien O'.

Damien O' was raised a Catholic. Although not particularly devout, he respects the faith of his youth and respects the religious beliefs of others. A Jesuit friend sends him *The Declaration on the Production and the Scientific and Therapeutic Use of Human Embryonic Stem Cells*, issued by the Pontifical Academy of Life Sciences. That document concludes that it is not "morally licit to produce and/or use living human embryos for the preparation of ES cells" and that it is not "morally licit to engage in so called 'therapeutic cloning' by producing cloned human embryos and then destroying them to produce ES cells." Damien's friend attaches a newspaper clipping quoting Pope John Paul II: "Experience is also showing how a tragic coarsening of consciences accompanies the assault on innocent human life in the womb . . . most recently, proposals for the creation for research purposes of human embryos, destined to destruction in the process."[2]

Damien O' is about to embark on his research. He has arranged to have a fertility clinic invite couples who do not need the fertilized embryos they have created to donate them to his research. Those embryos will be thawed and the ESTs dissected. Damien O' is thus engaging in "the use of a human embryo for the preparation of ES cells." Now, he wonders whether his conscience is, as the pope said, "coarsening." Also, one of his research fellows, an

American, tells him that her grandfather, a Southern Baptist minister, has written to her to express his dismay at her work. The leadership of the Southern Baptists has condemned stem cell research regardless of its purposes.

Damien O' need not worry about the legality of his work. His laboratory is in the United Kingdom where, since 1990, the Human Fertilization and Embryology Authority (HFEA) has effectively overseen the research and practice of assisted reproduction. The birth of Dolly the Sheep in Scotland inspired concern about extension of cloning to humans. At the same time, the therapeutic potential of EST research was acknowledged. HFEA regulations at first forbade creation of embryos for research, but in 2001, Parliament permitted creation of embryos by NT for research into potential therapy for serious diseases. The law represented what one member of the House of Lords described as a "sensible balance" between respect for the human embryo and relief from terrible disease.[3] HFEA was authorized to grant licenses to laboratories to proceed with stem cell research. Damien's laboratory is licensed.

He knows that in the United States things are quite different. There the debate about the cloning of babies, *reproductive cloning*, has spilled over into *therapeutic cloning*, cloning to develop treatments for disease. The verbal distinction and the prospect of a dramatically new form of medicine has not resolved the debate; it has stimulated it. Even the therapeutic value inherent in stem cells cannot justify the destruction of a human embryo, say the opponents. The debate is international. Some thirty nations have enacted legislation forbidding cloning for reproduction; a handful also prohibit therapeutic cloning. In 2004, a resolution was introduced in the United Nations to ban cloning for any reason; some sixty-two member nations are lined up behind the United States in support.

President George Bush devoted his first speech to the nation to stem cell research. In what was as much a moral sermon as a policy statement (one commentator noted that the president chose to appear before the nation for the first time in the role of a bioethicist!), he confessed his own beliefs, saying, "I believe that human life is a sacred gift from the Creator. I worry about a culture that devalues life and believe as your president that I have an important obligation to foster and encourage respect for life in America and throughout the world." He quoted a bioethicist as telling him, "[M]ake no mistake, that [five-day-old] cluster of cells is the same way you and I, and all the rest of us, started our lives. One goes with a heavy heart if we use these . . . because we are dealing with the seeds of the next generation." He then announced his decision to allow federal funds to support research only on existing stem cell lines, that is, stem cells that had already been obtained and cultured from frozen embryos donated by couples using in vitro fertilization. The destruction of embryos that produced these cells, he reasoned, had already taken place. He asserted that there were sixty such cell lines existing in laboratories around the world.[4]

The president named a bioethics council to monitor stem cell research and to recommend appropriate guidelines and regulations. Commentators generally believed that the council was stacked with conservative thinkers likely to follow the declared lead of its chair, Dr. Leon Kass, who had made his opposition to cloning and stem cell research clear in many articles. Commentators were wrong. While the council's report *Human Cloning and Human Dignity: An Ethical Inquiry*, released in July 2002, did unanimously reject cloning for purposes of producing children (as have all other international documents), its members split on the contentious issue of research cloning for therapeutic purposes. Rather than condemning the practice outright, the council could only muster sufficient votes for a moratorium on EST research, and that only by a ten to seven vote. The council's subsequent report, *Monitoring Stem Cell Research* (2004), did little more than reiterate the arguments on both sides of the debate and advise caution. Regardless of the relatively soft conclusion on EST research, the climate has not been favorable for such work in the United States. Congress continues efforts to ban it entirely; regulations surrounding funded research are so tightly drawn as to discourage researchers and their institutions from investing effort and money in it.

The ethical debate, particularly in the United States, has stuck on the question of embryo destruction. Equally troubling is the concomitant question of embryo creation and destruction for the purpose of research, as Korean scientists Woo Suk Hwang and Shin Yong Moon have done. Damien O' has finessed the first question by using embryos already created by couples seeking reproductive assistance. President Bush did the same by limiting research only to already existing cell lines and forbidding the creation of new ones. But these are temporizing solutions. Creation of embryos by NT offers many advantages to scientific exploration. Use of spare frozen embryos is limited by the relatively small number of these in existence around the world. Existing cell lines (of which there are far fewer than the president suggested) may not be able to proliferate and differentiate; they may be tainted by cells from the medium in which they are cultured (usually a plate of mouse cells); they do not represent the range of diseases needed for fruitful research. Thus, the question of creating and destroying human embryos remains alive.

The profound moral question of the status of the embryo lies beneath this question. We have already addressed this question in topic 7 on abortion. Those who uphold full moral status from fertilization cannot tolerate the destruction of the embryo; those who prefer the developmental thesis about moral status can justify various manipulations at various points in embryogenesis. Damien O', who was taught the Catholic doctrine that full human life begins at conception, is astonished to learn that some reputable Catholic theologians accept the developmental thesis and may permit intervention, even destruction, in the very early embryo, prior to implantation. He is also intrigued to learn that some Jewish scholars consider stem cell research morally obligatory: it contributes to the central Jewish moral tenet of protecting human life by the healing of disease.

Even if Damien O' is inclined toward the developmental position (it seems to him scientifically sensible), he must decide precisely how this embryo should be used and for what purposes. A term, *respect for the embryo*, has come into the debate. It is hard to decipher what it means. For those who take the "first moment" position, respect means that the embryo at conception deserves full protection for its life and full promotion of its flourishing. Those who espouse the developmental position also use the term to describe an attitude of reluctance to destroy embryonic life unless the destruction is justified by some greater good. Even then, other means of achieving that good should be preferred to using the embryo, if at all possible; if not, the least destructive course should be followed.

The ethical questions go beyond the balancing of the good of producing knowledge and therapy against the evil of destroying a developing human organism. Stem cells might be genetically manipulated in ways that not only eliminate disease but change human characteristics for eugenic purposes. Further, techniques to obtain ESTs require the utilization of human ova. This raises concerns about the exploitation of women to obtain ova and about the commodification or commercialization of human parts. Regenerative medicine might be so expensive that it would be available only to the well placed and wealthy, thus introducing another inequity into an already inequitable health care system. Inequity also may result from a biological fact: the histocompatibility genes that govern cell rejection differ significantly among persons of various ethnic backgrounds. Creation of a bank of cells could favor the majority population whose histocompatability genes are most widely represented; other populations might find it extremely difficult to gain access to cell therapy. Also, regenerative medicine may set society off on an ultimately futile quest for a world totally free of pain, disability, and disease. Finally, might a regenerative medicine, dependent on this consumptive use of human embryos, be ultimately a depreciation of human dignity rather than a benefit? These ethical questions, in addition to the status of the embryo, circle around the science of ESTs.

Proponents of stem cell research stress the duty to develop cures for devastating diseases. Several weeks before President Ronald Reagan died after a decade of mental decline from Alzheimer's disease, his wife, Nancy, made a public appeal in favor of stem cell research. Alzheimer's disease may not be a likely target for regenerative medicine in the near future, but other devastating neurological diseases such as Parkinson's disease are very likely targets. The prospect of regenerative therapy for these devastating conditions made the former first lady's appeal compelling. The most visible advocate for stem cell research was Christopher Reeve, Superman of the movies. Completely paralyzed after a fall from a horse, he appeared in his wheelchair, speaking with a mechanically amplified voice. The use of glial cells, derived from stem cells, holds promise for the neurological repair of devastating spinal injuries like his. (It should be noted that recent studies with adult stem cells have also shown some promise.)

Many more ravaging and fatal conditions await the promise of stem cell research, among them common diseases such as diabetes and the effects of heart attacks. Yet, those results are far off and may never eventuate. Can this speculative good serve as the justification for a palpable harm, the destruction of a living being, even at its earliest stage? Many commentators fear that so speculative a justification moves our society even further into a culture in which humans, even embryonic ones, are but means to ends.

On the other hand, this research is not wholly focused on creating restorative therapies, many of which may be far in the future or never eventuate. It has the more immediate purpose of gaining a deeper understanding of cell biology. The study of stem cells can unlock the most important secret of human growth and development, namely, the way in which, at the earliest stage of cellular existence, genes are activated and direct the production and folding of proteins that will guide each cell into a specific form of tissue. Access to ESTs opens the way toward exploration of fertilization and fetal development, spontaneous abortion, the origin of genetic defects, and the processes of many diseases, particularly, the deranged cellular processes of cancer cells. It can inform us about the efficacy and dangers of drugs. It promises a vast expansion and renovation of the scientific understanding of human biology and pathology. Thus, even if the expected therapies do not result, scientific progress will be made. Indeed, stem cells bear the seeds of a true scientific revolution in understanding health and disease, not unlike the advent of the germ theory in the nineteenth century. This, say proponents, is a great human good.

The ethics around stem cell research depend greatly on the confidence that one can place in various key assertions. These assertions flow from scientific observation, rational argument, faith claims, and political considerations. The scientific observations must be judged for their soundness. The rational arguments must be assessed for their consistency and use of evidence. The faith arguments must be evaluated on the moral authority of their sources in revelation and tradition. Political considerations must be viewed within the political philosophy of the nation.

Damien O' reflects on all of this. He believes that the science is reliable and genuinely promises treatments, although they remain far in the future. He accepts the developmental thesis of moral status as reasonable and is pleased to find some support from coreligionists on this point. He judges that a democratic society should respect but not consecrate the moral arguments of its citizens and that the view of the majority should prevail. He decides to proceed with his work in good conscience. Although, as a scientist, he might be thought biased toward research, he has also endeavored to make a conscientious and responsible judgment. His reflection could have come to another conclusion. Had he been convinced by the claim of human status for the embryo from the first moment, or more skeptical of the potential of ESTs, or more impressed by the potential of adult stem cells, or troubled by the possible injustices that might be caused by regenerative medicine, he might have judged otherwise. It is the purpose of bioethics to guide a conscientious person through these issues.

NOTES

1. *New York Times*, July 21, 2001, A9.
2. Pontifical Academy of Life Sciences, August 25, 2000, 6, 7, available at www .cin.org/docs/stem-cell research.html. "Remarks by John Paul," *New York Times*, July 24, 2001, A8.
3. *Lords Hansard*, January 22, 2001, columns 15–124.
4. G. W. Bush, "Federal Financing for Research with Embryonic Stem Cells," *New York Times*, August 10, 2001, A16.

BIBLIOGRAPHY

Bonnicksen, A. 2002. *Crafting a Cloning Policy. From Dolly to Stem Cells*. Washington, DC: Georgetown University Press.
Green, R. 2001. *The Human Embryo Research Debates: Bioethics in the Vortex of Controversy*. New York: Oxford University Press.
National Bioethics Advisory Commission. 1997. *Cloning Human Beings*. Washington, DC: U.S. Government Printing Office, at www.bioethics.gov.
National Bioethics Advisory Commission. 1999. *Ethical Issues in Stem Cell Research*. Washington, DC: U.S. Government Printing Office, at www.bioethics.gov.
National Institutes of Health. 2001. *Stem Cells: Scientific Progress and Future Research Directions*. Washington, DC: National Institutes of Health.

Nuffield Council on Bioethics. *Stem Cell Therapy: Ethical Issues*, at www.nuffield-bioethics.org.

President's Council on Bioethics. 2002. *Human Cloning and Human Dignity*. Washington, DC: U.S. Government Printing Office, at www.bioethics.gov.

President's Council on Bioethics. 2004. *Monitoring Stem Cell Research*. Washington, DC: President's Council, at www.bioethics.gov.

IV

THE WIDER WORLD
OF BIOETHICS

$\mathscr{P}$art IV of this book travels to and beyond the usual borders of bioethics. The usual borders are marked by the close interactions between several persons, often a physician and a patient or a researcher and a research subject. But those close interactions take place within a wider world. The most obvious wider world is the health care system itself. The health care system is not actually across the border of bioethics since bioethicists, especially in the last decade, have written frequently about it. Still, its large institutions and organizations, with their economics and politics, raise issues far beyond the interactions of individuals. Bioethics enters this wider world because those institutions and policies profoundly affect the shape and even the possibility of the private interactions. So, access to health care is the first topic in this section.

A next topic, cultural bioethics, recognizes that the issues of bioethics have appeared in many cultures. These issues sometimes result from the migration of people from other cultures into the Western world, where they encounter practices and values quite unfamiliar to them. More often, however, modern medical science and practice have moved into cultures with quite different views of life and death. Thus, the study of bioethics, which started in the United States and Britain, now flourishes in many nations. This topic will briefly review these indigenous bioethics.

The two final topics of this section, animal ethics and ecological ethics, are not usually found in bioethical books and journals. Still, an introduction to bioethics should introduce its readers to these topics. The "bio" in bioethics is a big prefix; it designates all life, not merely the life of the human organism. It certainly should not be confined to the damaged life treated by medicine. Concentration on clinical medicine and human biomedical science has led to the almost total neglect by bioethicists of much of the bioworld.

Animals other than humans dwell in one corner of bioethics, where they appear as guinea pigs, the objects of medical experiments. The environment of air, oceans and rivers, forests and fields is not considered at all in standard bioethics. A distinct discipline, ecology, considers to some extent the ethical issues associated with the preservation of the environment. Still, it is worth asking whether the ethical principles of bioethics are meaningful in these boundary matters.

There is a second reason to end this book with these topics. It is an act of homage to the man who invented the word "bioethics" itself, the biomedical research scientist Van Rensselaer Potter. When he introduced the word in 1970, he intended it to name "a new discipline that combines biological knowledge with a knowledge of human value systems." This new science was to identify and promote an optimum changing environment and an optimum human adaptation within that environment so as to sustain and improve living. Bioethics, for Potter, was the study of *bios* in its largest sense: the entirety of life. He aimed to understand what modern environmental scientists call the biosphere and to explore how human action best fits into and preserves it. Unfortunately, Potter was unable to construct the "new science" in a form that appealed widely. Quickly, the word that he created was usurped by medicine and the biomedical sciences. It may be time to attend again to his call for a "science of survival" in which we come to "respect the fragile web of life and . . . broaden . . . knowledge to include the nature of man and his relation to the biological and physical worlds."[1]

So, this final part calls out the animals and explores the environment as a larger bioethics, sensitive to the biosphere. Since both topics are very large, I will only explore them at the margins, where they touch some of the more familiar questions of bioethics.

NOTE

1. V. Potter, *Bioethics: Bridge to the Future* (Englewood Cliffs, NJ: Prentice Hall, 1971), 2, 4.

• *Topic 12* •

Bioethics and the Health Care System

"Patients Excluded from Life-Saving Treatment"

In 1962, Dr. Belding Scribner of the University of Washington in Seattle had an ingenious idea for the treatment of serious kidney disease. A small plastic tube, sewn into the vein and artery of the wrist, might allow a patient's entire blood supply to be drained out, passed through a "washing machine," and run back into the patient's body. This "dialysis" would cleanse the blood of poisons accumulated when the patient's kidneys were unable to do this vital job. The "washing machine" was, in effect, an artificial kidney. Dr. Scribner adapted a technique that had been invented some twenty years earlier so that it could be used on a continuous basis for persons with end-stage kidney disease. These persons would die within a few months of diagnosis; now they could live for years with regular weekly attachment to the dialysis machine. This was hailed as a medical miracle: it was the first, truly life-sustaining medical technology. But it posed a problem: many more patients needed the treatment than Dr. Scribner's small unit could provide. A committee of anonymous laypersons was formed to choose those from among medically suitable candidates who would be admitted. In a television documentary about this program, one of the chosen is asked, "What happened to the others." He answers, "They died."

DR. GAWANDE'S VISIT HOME

Dr. Atul Gawande, an American-educated surgeon, returned to his ancestral home, Nanded, India, to serve as a visiting surgeon. He found a city hospital

141

that served fourteen hundred villages and 2.3 million people with five hundred beds, three operating rooms, and nine general surgeons. Almost none of these 2.3 million people had health insurance. The few private hospitals were tiny and far too expensive for the ordinary Indian. Yet, Dr. Gawande's medical colleagues unhesitatingly stated that they would use those private facilities for themselves and their families.[1]

These are two stories about the scarcity of health care resources. In the first, particular patients, with names and addresses, families and friends, are selected to receive a life-sustaining treatment. This story occasioned the article mentioned at the very beginning of this book, "Who Lives? Who Dies? Who Decides?" In the second story, a health care system is stretched to capacity, without adequate funds and too expensive for many who need its services. Here, the Who lives? Who dies? question may also be asked but the fortunate and unfortunate are not identified as individual persons. They are statistics: a certain percentage of sick who need care will not receive it. Most of these statistics represent persons who never reach a doctor or the doors of a hospital. Yet, they live or die due to the scarcity of health resources.

Scarcity of health resources has many causes: the socioeconomic level of the country, the form and financing of the health care system, competition between health care and other social needs, costly medical innovations, excessive profits for pharmaceutical companies, growing numbers of senior persons who use health care more frequently, discrimination that makes care scarce for certain classes and racial groups, and political machinations. The paucity and poverty of Indian health care arises principally from the general state of socioeconomic development in that vast nation; the restrictions of the American, Canadian, and British systems reflect political and economic policy in wealthy nations. In the United States in particular, the prevalence of a market system of medicine, supplemented by federal and state assistance for the elderly and the indigent, allows medical service to "follow the money." In 2003, 43.6 million Americans, 15.2 percent of the population, had no health insurance; most of these were employed persons whose employer did not provide insurance and who fell into an income category making them ineligible for state supported insurance and incapable of buying private insurance.

"The American health care system is characterized by both feast and famine: it leads the world in delivering high tech medical miracles but leaves 45 million people uninsured."[2] Feast or famine is an ambiguous metaphor. In emphasizing that many Americans enjoy an abundance of excellent care, while many others have very restricted access, it fails to reveal that in large part, the famine is caused by the feast. In the United States, continual innovation in medical technology and treatments creates market demand from doctors, patients, and hospitals. Replacement of body parts, from hearts to hips; drugs for mental distress, from serious psychoses to mild mood disorders; refined diagnostic machines that can quickly spot fractures, tumors, or infections; complex pharmaceutical regimens for patients with chronic diseases—all of these, to name but a few, make American medicine the most expensive in the world. And their lifesaving and life-improving capabilities flow largely to those who can afford to pay for them (these benefits do come to the poor fortunate enough to have access to public health care systems, but the public pays for them).

The American feast for some, with its attendant famine for others, is very different from the Indian health care famine that Dr. Gawande encountered. The economies of developing nations are beset by constraints and shortages in all basic needs. Health care struggles along with food production and distribution, water supply, sewage treatment, availability of subsistence jobs, and every other human need. The problem of scarcity in health care must be addressed in terms of very different settings and causal factors.

Scarcity is the setting for a practical problem: how are scarce resources to be distributed among all who need them? This is not merely a practical problem, solvable by good planning. It is an ethical problem: what are the standards for selection? Are those standards fair and just? The failure of the American flu vaccine supply in 2004 provides a clear example. Priority groups for vaccination, such as the elderly, persons with chronic illnesses, pregnant women, all children under two, and health care workers, amounted to 98 million people; 41 million doses of vaccine were available. The Centers for Disease Control appointed a panel of bioethicists to advise on fair allocation.[3] Should high-risk children be vaccinated before high-risk adults? Should the elderly be vaccinated before the chronically ill? Should all such criteria be considered invidious and a lottery established? This is a clear and obvious example of the ethical problem of fair allocation; the bioethicists who debate the questions are familiar with the arguments, as we shall see below, and struggle to apply familiar principles to this new problem. But the problem becomes far more complex outside of settings like epidemics, where needs can be estimated and the resources counted.

In recent times, as medicine has become more technological and institutional, the problem of justice has become a central one. Not long ago, a visit to the doctor ended with some sage advice and a simple, relatively inexpensive prescription. Today, that meeting may generate costly tests, which may propel the patient into a hospital, a complex institution built to accommodate elaborate technology and intensive procedures. Doctors and nurses are now surrounded by other highly trained personnel who manage the technology. The hospital itself is a massive bureaucracy with arcane financing, flowing from government programs and private insurers, from bond issues, loans, donations, and patients' pockets. Medical-supply industries and pharmaceutical manufacturers constantly develop new devices and drugs and aggressively market them. Legal regulations abound, and legal liability for malpractice is a constant threat. In American medicine, the profit motive is everywhere. In other countries, where national health care schemes have mitigated the profit motive, other influences, such as public-financing constraints and government control, dominate the system. The complexity of modern health care distributes not only the good of health care but also the goods of money and influence across populations of patients, doctors, administrators, politicians, and investors. The question of whether this complex system of distribution can meet any standard of justice is a daunting one.

Dr. Scribner's Seattle Dialysis Center came up with its solution to the problem of scarcity. Many patients needed the service; the service was limited. The limits were set because there was but one center in the United States and a handful of doctors and nurses able to manage the delicate procedure. Also, the cost was higher than many patients could pay ($10,000 per year in 1962), and insurance was reluctant to reimburse this innovative technique. Most problematic was the fact that dialysis had to be continued for the remaining life of the patient. Thus, the population of patients needing treatment grew year after year.

Dr. Scribner's story illustrates the problem of justice at its most painful level, the need of particular patients for a scarce resource. Although dedicated to saving his own sick patients, he quickly realized that his attempt to save individual lives thrust his work into the larger dimension of health policy. An admissions and policy committee was created to deal with the problem of selecting patients for the nine-bed clinic. Beyond that clinic, twenty thousand persons diagnosed each year with end-stage renal disease were waiting. The committee sat down monthly with some ten medical folders of patients judged medically suitable for dialysis; they chose one or two out of the stack to fill any spot that had become available. They struggled to come up with reasonable, fair criteria: parents of young children were preferred to persons without dependants, younger persons to older, employed to unemployed. The further they went with this search for reasonable criteria, the more perplexed they became. Should a churchgoer be chosen over a nonchurchgoer, a voter over a nonvoter? Still, perplexed as they were, they had to choose.

THE ETHICAL ARGUMENTS

Early bioethicists were fascinated by the problem posed by the Seattle Committee: is there an ethical way to select patients for life or death? The problem pitted utilitarian ethics against egalitarian ethics. Egalitarians commend random selection as the only mechanism consonant with the dignity and equality of all candidates. Patients should be selected by a lottery blind to their individual characteristic. Utilitarians demand selection of those whose lives contribute to society. These two positions rest on two distinct foundations for moral judgment. Utilitarians rely on social utility, that is, the achievement of the greater good for the greater number in a society. Egalitarians assert the absolute moral claim of each person to basic human goods, such as life and liberty, and repudiate judgments of comparative social worth.

One Utilitarian ethicist writes, "Society 'invests' a scarce resource in one person as against another and is thus entitled to look to the probable prospective 'return' on its investment." This principle of social utility suggests certain criteria for selecting (or excluding) entire groups for a scarce resource— criteria that will maximize society's return on its investment. The life expectancy of the candidates, their family roles and responsibilities, their work history, their contributions to society, and the prospect of future contributions are all relevant to their candidacy. These selection criteria involve valuing each candidate for his or her "social worth." Future contributions and past service are particularly valued. The philosopher acknowledges that such judgments are difficult, yet affirms that "such distasteful problems must be faced, since a failure to choose some is tantamount to sentencing all. Unpleasant choices are intrinsic to the problem of selection." This philosopher endorses the utilitarian approach of the Seattle selection committee, where rough calculations of social worth seemed to play so large a role.[4]

Several theological bioethicists have endorsed the Egalitarian argument. They argue that the dignity of each person is the primary moral criterion. Random selection honors the dignity of each person. Society would more readily accept random selection as fair over an assessment of the personal worth of individuals, which can favor the wealthy, the well connected, and the socially acceptable. The utilitarian approach is neither feasible nor justifiable. It is not feasible because it is impossible to quantify and compare the values that should be counted in assessing social worth. It is not justifiable because, as one author writes, "the utilitarian approach would, in effect, reduce the person to his social role. . . . A person's transcendence, his dignity as a person . . . cannot be reduced to his past or future contribution to society." That dignity and transcendence "can be protected and witnessed to by a recognition of his equal right to be saved." The only mechanism consistent with this recognition is a lottery in which each person has an equal opportunity to be saved.[5]

One article criticizes mercilessly the "prejudices and mindless clichés that pollute the [Seattle] committee's deliberations . . . the bourgeoisie sparing the bourgeoisie . . . [ruling out] the creative non-conformists, who rub the bourgeoisie the wrong way but who historically have contributed so much to the making of America. The Pacific Northwest is no place for a Henry David Thoreau with bad kidneys." Although society does evaluate persons in many, often biased ways, in the matter at hand—the provision of a lifesaving resource—evaluation, these authors assert, approaches the impossible. The only way to avoid evaluation is by lottery or by the first come, first serve rule.[6]

Far from seeing a human lottery as appropriate to human dignity, some ethicists have been repelled by the idea. Joseph Fletcher, a frank utilitarian, called a lottery "literally irresponsible, a rejection of the burden, refusal to be rational." A lottery poses many practical difficulties. It requires that a group gather before lots can be drawn, a situation that is unrealistic because patients appear serially with an urgent need for help. Lotteries can be rigged and, in matters of such import, are likely to be. Even a queue can be "jumped" by those who have knowledge and power. Some authors doubt that random selection would alleviate anxiety, and several authors distinguish between the "natural" sorts of random selection, such as the first come, first serve rule, and artificial ones, such as lotteries. All systems of random selection make it possible for socially disreputable and dangerous persons to be the lucky winners of the gift of life, a prospect that critics of the lottery find unpalatable but proponents consider the price of fairness. This vigorous debate over selection of patients for a scarce resource came to be called the *microallocation problem*, picking out the fortunate few from the many needy at the point of service. This was a modern version of the old medical triage (said to have been devised by Napoleon's medical corps), where battlefield surgeons selected out of the many wounded those they could repair most effectively and rush back to battle.

The five bioethicists chosen to sit on the Centers for Disease Control panel on fair allocation of scarce flu vaccine will know the story of the Seattle case and the large literature that surrounds it. Their task will be to apply those lessons to the conditions of scarcity posed by the catastrophic failure of the American flu-vaccine supply system. (In the end, a sufficient supply of vaccine was obtained so that a rationing system was not needed on a national scale.)

UNIVERSAL ACCESS TO HEALTH SERVICES

Dr. Gawande's visit to his Indian homeland reveals another sort of health care scarcity. A vast population of persons with marginal economic means bring their illnesses and injuries to a small, stressed, and underfunded health care system. Many never get in the door. In the past, these persons would have sought the treatments of traditional ayurvedic medicine provided by practitioners dwelling in their villages. They would have been cared for at home by family. Now they seek the services of technologically trained physicians and technologically equipped hospitals. It is this form of health care that is unavailable to so many Indian citizens.

A much larger problem than the selection of individual patients looms over technological medicine. At the dawn of bioethics, medical services were still provided as a cottage industry. Patients sought the attention of physicians in their offices and surgeries. They were admitted to private and community hospitals for operations and extended care. Patients paid doctors out of their pocket or savings. The unpredictable advent of illness often made it difficult to pay for care, so various insurance schemes helped pay the doctor's bill. In the United States, insurance was usually provided by commercial insurers and made available in association with one's employment. The poor were accommodated in public hospitals, and doctors provided some "charity care" in accord with ancient tenets of medical ethics. In that simpler medical world, there was little concern about equality.

In Great Britain after World War II, the Labor government achieved a remarkable revolution in health services. It made equality of access a major goal. A deeply rooted private practice system was transformed into the National Health System (NHS), in which health workers became government employees and hospitals, including even the great teaching hospitals, became government institutions. The principles of the NHS were universality (care was provided to all, regardless of age, class, sex, or religion), comprehensiveness (a full range of care was provided), and free access (no patient paid for care received). In the United States, the private-practice system prevailed, although a public insurance system partially covered the elderly (Medicare) and the indigent (Medicaid). It was anticipated that a sort of rough equality could be achieved by these policies.

The new medical technologies arrived in these settings, and strains soon appeared. Novel diagnostic techniques, such as magnetic resonance imaging (MRI), could perform wonders in detecting disease yet were very expensive. Expanded capacity to detect and treat disease pressured the systems into more complex forms of care, in which increasing numbers of specialists and services became involved in a case. A growing population of elderly persons had health needs that had to be met. The complexity raised costs and also offered opportunity for profit that had never been present in health care.

Concern about access to all medical treatment, not only to the expensive and "exotic" forms, became a national issue in the United States and Great Britain. The glowing expectations that the NHS and Medicare and Medicaid would bring the benefits of the new medicine to all citizens were beginning to fade. The cost of medical care and the proportion of the national product devoted to its financing became a major public concern. The costs of health care were increasing faster than costs in the general economy. Government and taxpayers began to feel the burden of public programs. As costs rose, access diminished. The NHS responded to scarcity by a form of implicit rationing, namely, extending the waiting time to be seen and to receive certain procedures. The Canadian system responded by economizing on expensive technological devices, such as MRIs. The American system, being so diverse, responded in diverse ways. Medicare and Medicaid reduced doctors' payments; managed care systems were instituted by organizations that paid for care. These systems, ironically called health maintenance organizations (HMOs), placed restrictions on doctors' use of tests, hospitalization, and costly drugs and on the time a doctor could spend with a patient.

The problem of inadequate access to health care is an economic or political problem. It is equally an ethical problem. Bioethicists began to take up this *macroallocation problem*, seeking criteria for a just allocation of resources across an entire health system. This is a problem of justice rather than fairness, as is the microallocation problem. Fairness regulates dealings with individuals; justice proposes institutional structures that make possible fair dealings. Justice, in its traditional definition, requires that social burdens and benefits be distributed according to (1) merit, (2) contribution, (3) market supply and demand, (4) need, and (5) similar treatment of similar cases. Bioethicists recognized that the first three criteria do not suit the nature of the social good that health and health care are; the latter two criteria are the proper ones to analyze justice in health care.[7] Even when need and equality are acknowledged as the primary criteria for justice, determining what constitutes need, how serious it is in comparison with other needs, and how it is distinguished from preferences and desires leaves many complex questions.

Social justice discussions in Western society frequently invoke the important philosophical and political notion of rights. The right to health care became a popular slogan. Yet, even philosophers who were dedicated to equity and fairness in health care worried that the strong endorsement of a positive right to health care would require dedication of unlimited resources to the health benefits of individuals. Such a right would rule out comparisons between health goods and other social goods, such as education, environmental protection, and defense. Even when these thinkers cautiously approved the idea of a right to health care, they denied that any particular health care intervention, such as cardiac transplantation or artificial heart implantation, must be provided as a matter of right to every individual needing such an intervention, even if it is lifesaving. Even a right to health care in general might require some sort of restrictive policies about access or, in terms unpalatable to many commentators, "rationing" of health care. However, the lifesaving nature of many medical interventions seems to obstruct all efforts to implement restrictive policy. The rational judgment that expensive lifesaving interventions should be rationed counters a strong psychological and social imperative to save those threatened by death.

One analysis of justice in health care has become the starting point for much subsequent discussion. This analysis adapts to health care the theory of justice elaborated by Harvard philosopher John Rawls. Rawls formulated an innovative version of the social contract, a common theme in political philosophy. He imagined that society comes into being when a collection of rational individuals contract to create social institutions behind "a veil of ignorance," which hides from their view the social status and class, intelligence, strength, and talents that each one might enjoy once the society based upon their contract comes into being. They must determine the principles that will govern their institutions and the distributions of social goods without knowing whether they will be among the better or worse off members of the society. Their contract will, then, specify two principles: "first, each person is to have an equal right to the most extensive liberty compatible with a similar liberty for others and, second, social and economic inequalities are to be arranged so that they are both (a) reasonably expected to be to everyone's advantage, and (b) attached to positions and offices open to all."[8]

Bioethicist Norman Daniels imported Rawls's thesis into a theory of justice about the social good of health care. He seeks philosophically sound answers to such questions as: What sort of a social good is health care? Are there social obligations to provide health care? What inequalities in its distribution are morally acceptable? What limits do individual liberties of physicians and patients place on just distribution of care? Daniels recognizes that health care is an enormously complex enterprise, ranging from recommending aspirin for headaches to transplanting hearts, from nursing care to neurosurgery, and from health education to accident prevention. He sees in that complexity one fundamental aim, the preservation of *normal species functioning* that is impaired by illness and disability. Normal species functioning comprises the activities most widely associated with being human: thinking and communicating, mobility and control, engagement in social activities, and the like. When normal species functioning at the biological and social levels is impaired, individuals are hindered from pursuing their "plans of life" and thus denied equal opportunity to enjoy the benefits of social life. Health and health care are linked to the primary social good of opportunity. The institutions that deliver health care and the social policies that structure those institutions are just and fair when they are designed to provide to each individual "a fair share of the normal opportunity range for their society at each stage of their life."[9]

That opportunity range, Daniels insists, extends over the full lifetime of individuals. Rational persons choosing the principles of fair health care behind "the veil of ignorance," he believes, would assure that they had available to themselves the kind of health care that would support their opportunities at various stages of life. They would not judge it unfair to be denied heart transplants or renal dialysis as elderly persons if they had enjoyed the full range of services that supported health during their youth and middle age. Daniels's key to the allocation problem is not rationing of specific technologies or services but their distribution through those ranges of opportunity in which they can most effectively sustain normal species functioning. Although Daniels's account of justice in health care is not without its critics, it has greatly advanced the discussion and served as a theoretically articulate basis for the escalating debate over access to health care.

A few bioethicists, such as the pioneer Dan Callahan, have ruminated about the roots of the allocation problem as we experience it in modern America. To Callahan, it is obvious that the problem arises from our cultural inability to acknowledge limits to life and to face the reality of death. The problem of scarcity in health care is, at bottom, a problem of inappropriate human priorities in an individualistic society. Individuals and medicine must realign priorities, directing attention to the health of the young rather than the elderly and devoting technical skills to the relief of suffering rather than conquest of death. Callahan's telling insights are a small voice in a very loud debate, but their echo can be heard in a report of the President's Council on Bioethics, *Beyond Therapy: Biotechnology and the Pursuit of Happiness* (2003). The council notes that the use of biotechnology "in order to try to satisfy deep and familiar human desires: for better children, superior performance, ageless bodies, and happy souls . . . present[s] us with profound and highly consequential ethical challenges and choices."[10]

During the 1990s, the word "rationing," previously shunned, entered the health care debate. The idea that a prosperous society would deliberately deprive sick persons of care had seemed almost obscene. Now, it became obvious that it was not enough merely to devise fair systems for selecting patients; it was necessary to devise institutional structures and rules that would limit the seemingly inexhaustible demands for medical care by increasingly needy populations. Case after case appeared. For example, the left-ventricular assist device (LVAD) was invented to support a failing heart until a heart transplant could be obtained; it was called "bridge to transplant." LVAD has recently been shown to extend life by some three months, in comparison with best medical management, for patients who are ineligible for transplant due to age or other medical complications. This is named, somewhat grimly, *destination therapy*. Some two hundred thousand patients per year could benefit from implantation of this device.

Many health economists would apply to this problem the form of analysis called *quality adjusted life years* (QALYs): one QALY equals one year of life without disability. A year of life with some disability equals a QALY less than one. An analysis of the use of LVAD for this category of patient shows a benefit of 0.7 QALYs, at a cost of $988,122, for a single patient. This calculation, multiplied by the number of possible patients, has a major impact on health care and health costs with little extension of life. But, some will say, it's life, and if the patient chooses it, he or she should have it. Others respond that a just and fair health care system must place limits on autonomy. Daniels's thesis about allocation of health resources over a lifetime and for the purpose of maintaining normal species function casts suspicion on the ethical wisdom of LVAD for destination therapy.

The state of Oregon launched the most vigorous attack on inequality in American health care. In 1994, the state legislature set up a health services commission charged with making "a list of health services ranked by priority from the most important to the least important, representing the comparative benefits of each service to the entire population to be served (considering clinical effectiveness and cost effectiveness)." The "population to be served" comprised the most impoverished Oregonians, who could not afford private insurance and were dependent on the state-funded Medicaid program. The objective was to conserve funds by rationing services to this population, but the conservation of funds was to be used to spread coverage more widely across this same population. The commission analyzed the medical literature on efficacy and on cost (often a very deficient literature), consulted bioethicists, held many community meetings, and at last, issued a list of 743 condition/treatment pairs that started with "severe or moderate brain injury with hematoma, edema and loss of consciousness" and ended with "radial keratotomy for disorders of refraction (of the eye)." It was left to the legislature to determine how far down that list the state's annual budget could fund procedures. In 1999, they put the cutoff at number 566, "medical or surgical treatment of urinary incontinence." An infant born with the fatal hypoplastic left-heart system would be deprived of number 567, a difficult and often ineffective but sometimes lifesaving surgery.

The list generated heated discussion. For many it was a dramatic advance in attempting to meld the dual problems of cost and fairness; for others, it was an example of depriving the already deprived of many needed procedures. Yet, the Oregon experiment has spread insurance coverage: between 1990 and 2000, the numbers of Oregonians without coverage decreased from 18 to 11 percent. The list is not the only element behind this improvement: many other modifications in health policy and practice have also been implemented. The experiment demonstrates that the bioethical principles of fairness and justice in health care require the complex collaboration of politicians, the professions, and the public. This is bioethics in practice.[11]

Justice in health care became one of the central questions of bioethics in the 1990s. American bioethicists participated vigorously in the political debates about health reform. It is painfully obvious that the best theoretical solutions, meeting high standards of justice, must be plunged into the complex of science, business, economics, and politics that constitutes modern health care.

NOTES

1. *New York Times*, December 21, 2003, Week in Review, 5.

2. Steve Lohr, "Is Kaiser the Future of American Health Care?" *New York Times*, October 31, 2004, 3, 4

3. D. Ricks, "Flu Shot Shortage," *Newsday* (October 31, 2004).

4. N. Rescher, "The Allocation of Exotic Medical Lifesaving Therapy," *Ethics* 79 (1967): 173–86.

5. J. Childress, "Who Shall Live When Not All Can Live?" *Soundings*, 53 (1970): 339–55.

6. D. Sanders and J. Dukeminier, "Medical Advance and Legal Lag: Hemodialysis and Kidney Transplantation," *UCLA Law Review* 15 (1968): 366–80.

7. G. Outka, "Social Justice and Equal Access to Health Care," *Journal of Religious Ethics* 2 (1974): 11–32.

8. J. Rawls, *A Theory of Justice* (Cambridge, MA: Harvard University Press, 1971).

9. N. Daniels, *Just Health Care* (New York: Cambridge University Press, 1985).

10. The President's Council on Bioethics, *Beyond Therapy: Biotechnology and the Pursuit of Happiness* (Washington, DC: Government Printing Office, 2002), available at www.bioethics.gov.

11. Office of Oregon Health Policy and Research, at www.ohppr.state.or.us.

BIBLIOGRAPHY

Beauchamp, T., and J. Childress. 2001. *Principles of Biomedical Ethics*, ch. 6. New York: Oxford University Press.

Callahan, D. 1987. *Setting Limits: Medical Goals in an Aging Society*. New York: Simon & Schuster.

Callahan, D. 1995. *What Kind of Life?* Washington, DC: Georgetown University Press.

Daniels, N. 1985. *Just Health Care*. New York: Cambridge University Press.

Danis, M., C. Clancy, and L. Churchill, eds. 2002. *Ethical Dimensions of Health Care*. New York: Oxford University Press.

Morreim, E. 1995. *Balancing Act: The New Medical Ethics of Medicine's New Economics*. Washington, DC: Georgetown University Press.

Reich, W., ed. 1995. "Health Care Financing," "Health Care Resources, Allocation of," and "Health Policy," *Encyclopedia of Bioethics*. New York: Macmillan.

Rhodes, R., M. Battin, and A. Silvers. 2001. *Medicine and Social Justice*. New York: Oxford University Press.

• *Topic 13* •

Cultural Bioethics

"Doctors Troubled by Immigrant Patients"

$\mathcal{M}$rs. Chu is an eighty-seven-year-old woman recently brought by her children from Taiwan to California. She does not speak English but is friendly and active. She has recently been ill, and doctors have diagnosed advanced ovarian cancer. Her two sons strongly object to telling their mother the diagnosis. They say, "This is not done in our culture." Vietnamese Hmong parents, relocated to Idaho, are reported to Child Protective Services by a neighbor, who accuses them of abusing their children by putting heated coins on their skin. The parents explain that this is a traditional manner of curing childhood ailments. A gynecologist serving a clinic in East London sees many Somalian and Ethiopian women with genitourinary problems due to the traditional practice of clitoridectomy. Today, her first patient is a twelve-year-old girl with serious infection after being mutilated by a traditional practitioner. The girl's mother vigorously defends the practice as holy and good for women. In all these cases, cultural traditions have crossed borders. In each case, the justification arises from a tradition not shared by the host culture.

Although this book has discussed bioethical matters very largely within American and British borders, bioethics breaks across borders. It has become an international interest. Many nations now sustain active bioethical programs. Scholars from Scandinavia to South Africa, from Santiago to Singapore, communicate at meetings and in many journals. Many nations have standing government bodies to deal with bioethical issues. The European Community has a bioethics commission that has studied many of the topics reviewed in this book; the European Bioethics Convention (1996) of the Council of Europe states the fundamental rights of human beings in bio-

154

science and medicine. UNESCO has the Division of Ethics of Science and Technology. An Asian bioethics society gathers scholars from Japan, China, India, Thailand, and other nations. Centers for the study of bioethics have opened in Argentina and Chile, and courses exist across Latin America. The International Society for Bioethics meets biannually.

As these voices have entered the conversation, different views on the issues emerge. European bioethicists tend to characterize the principles of bioethics differently than do Americans: they list, for example, dignity, integrity, vulnerability, and subsidarity, along with autonomy. They tend to interpret autonomy in a Kantian rather than Millsian fashion: autonomy is the capacity to act in accord with moral reason rather than the unimpeded liberty to act as one chooses. Issues are seen differently. In Japan, heart transplantation was long rejected as incompatible with cultural attitudes. In the European Community, bioethicists, still mindful of Nazi eugenics, have been particularly cautious about genetics research. Although Israel is a secular nation, the influence of rabbinic prohibitions discourages termination of artificial life support. Developing countries have different priorities in health care than countries where investment in health care is high. The "internationalizing" of epidemics due to easy and extensive travel means that the ethics of dealing with infectious disease (which often require restrictive preventive measures) must also be international, incorporating the values of various cultures. Thus, international bioethics reveals a wide and diverse scope of issues.

However, international bioethics also reveals a classical ethical problem: ethical relativism. Does the fact of different cultural norms for ethical behavior imply that all ethical norms are relative to the cultures in which they are found and are valid only in that time and place? Does it imply that there are no universal ethical norms that cross the borders of culture, tradition, and history? This has long been a perplexing problem in moral philosophy, and it reappears in modern bioethics. It appears most acutely when persons from one cultural tradition encounter the health care of another culture.

Bioethicists discuss both the broad differences between cultures and the particular problems that arise when the moral norms of one culture conflict with those of another. Interest in the broad differences is mainly descriptive: How do Italians view the authority of physicians? What do Theravada Buddhists think about life support technology? Do Muslims permit abortion? When persons from these cultures answer such questions, outsiders can comprehend, even if they might not approve. The problems of conflict are often viewed as practical problems that might be managed by changes in strategy, by accommodation, by education. Thus, the conflict about Mrs. Chu's right to know her diagnosis might be negotiated by asking her whether she is willing to allow her family to guide her care. This strategy would uphold both the

Western importance of autonomy and informed consent and the Chinese respect for elders and reticence.

Bioethicists have rarely plunged into the deep philosophical waters of ethical relativism on which these descriptive and practical problems float. Yet, when faced with certain practices, bemused curiosity, toleration, or mild disapproval seems hardly enough. Certainly, many judge that it is not enough to deplore genital mutilation but imperative to eradicate it, regardless of its acceptance in certain cultures. Should not infanticide be stopped and punished, regardless of its cultural toleration? Even if unprotected sex is the cultural norm, should it not be criticized when lethal infectious disease is transmitted thereby? It would be unusual for even the most liberal Western person to tolerate these practices on the grounds that morality is relative, in other words, that what each person or each culture judges right is in fact right for that person or culture.

Philosophers have argued forever about moral relativity. It is obvious to any observer that peoples in different places have different ways and values. It should also be obvious, philosophers point out, that it is illogical to infer from these differences that any form of moral belief is as valid as any other. The fact of difference does not prove the validity of the different practices. That proof, if there be one, depends on a careful delineation of the issue and an even more careful assessment of the arguments pro and con. The delineation attempts to describe accurately the practices, to distinguish between custom and morality, to clarify the explanations and reasons given for certain practices, and to explore their historical origins and place within the setting of culture, religion, law, and economics. Once these clarifications are made, some apparent differences disappear, and others seem innocuous. Indeed, many commentators claim that beneath the differences, certain common moral universals can be glimpsed.

The prohibitions against unprovoked killing of persons, lying, and breaking of promises seem to be essential rules to establish trust between people and to allow them to deal with each other. Thus, if any ethical rules are universal, found in all human societies, these basic ones are among them. Many other ethical rules appear in quite different forms and with different degrees of emphasis but, on examination, also seem to serve the essential function of holding a society together. In the words of philosopher G. J. Warnock, ethics "ameliorates the human predicament." Thus, ethical rules about relations between the sexes appear very differently in different cultures, but essentially they serve to support the essential task of procreating and educating the young of the society.

These purported moral universals are not easy to express. In Anglo-American bioethics, the principle of respect for autonomy has, to our ears, the ring of universality. It is rooted in philosophical reflections about human nature and rationality. Yet, it does not ring so true in many cultures. While Confucianism, for example, inculcates a deep respect for persons, it does not include in that concept any particular deference to the choices and preferences of individuals, as does our concept of respect for autonomy. In many cultures, personal autonomy is surrounded, almost to invisibility, with the preeminence of family and community. Yet, even where this is so, concern about the safety, welfare, and dignity of individuals remain constants. The wishes of individuals may be subordinated to a common good, but the individual will still be cherished and honored, and the individual will flourish within the community. This is clearly a different view of our bioethical principle; yet, a basic moral affirmation about the value of persons remains. Indeed, it will often surface when some group begins to feel a radical deprivation of personhood. Women in some traditional societies affirm a right to be educated; "untouchables" claim political and economic rights. The idea of fundamental human rights, so widely accepted internationally, requires some such universality of principle. Indeed, advocacy for human rights, particularly in the realm of health, motivates such organizations as Doctors without Borders. These physicians, who bring their medical skills anywhere, even to the most dangerous places, are not bioethicists, but their work manifests the bioethical principles of respect for persons, beneficence, and justice.

Still, the philosophical problem of relativism remains: is it possible to affirm that ethical practices of a certain sort are universally right or wrong? Put differently, is it legitimate to criticize and condemn the moral standards of other cultures or to attempt to eradicate or reform them? Philosophers who answer in the affirmative often suggest that a negative answer involves an inherent contradiction. If someone claims, they say, that all moral practices are valid for those who practice them and that it is wrong to condemn such practices, that person is making a moral judgment that he or she believes universally valid. If proponents of moral relativism were true to their doctrine, they would refrain even from saying that we must tolerate or respect the moral beliefs of others. Such a statement is empty since anyone hearing it can respond, "That is just your opinion." This inherent contradiction does not prove that there are universal moral norms; it does show that it is difficult to demonstrate that there are none.

In addition to these philosophical problems about intercultural bioethics, there are sociopolitical ones. The economic and political differences between nations influence the forms of health care available to the people and also the prevalence of disease and disability. The AIDS crisis in sub-Saharan Africa has made this most visible. In a part of the world that supports 10 percent of the world's population, dwell 70 percent of persons infected with HIV.

Many of its countries are devastated as thousands of its young people die and thousands are orphaned. Yet, general health care is inadequate, political leadership is weak, and the costs of those drugs that are now common in the West are prohibitive. Local traditions of family, sexuality, and religion impede health education.

Research to develop vaccines and antiviral drugs is imperative; yet, research protocols implemented in those countries have been highly criticized as exploitive. International policies have been developed by many organizations. They generally assert that researchers who develop new treatments using persons in developing nations as subjects should ensure that the results of this research are made reasonably available to the people of those nations. This seems an unrealistic standard to many. Recently, the *principle of fair benefits* has been suggested: researchers must design research so that, in exchange for the participation of subjects, some valuable and useful benefit resulting from the research (not necessarily a new product) is left with the nation where the research was conducted. For example, researchers who study the sociological effects of introducing antiretroviral drugs for HIV/AIDS may contribute to a more effective health policy on the use of these drugs as a public health measure. Bioethics must continue to explore the dimensions of international justice in health care and research.

The bioethical discussion that has opened between cultures not only reveals differences; it also broadens understanding. Indeed, it sometimes imports ideas into cultures where persons are seeking them. One bioethicist who has taken seriously the problem of cultural relativism, Prof. Ruth Macklin, observes that often, in discussions with persons in other cultures, her explanation of a Western value, such as the principle of autonomy, while foreign to that culture, inspires people to formulate their own arguments against some traditional custom, such as genital mutilation or subordination of wives to their husbands, that they are seeking to change. She points out that such Western practices as informed consent for treatment and for research are quickly understood in authoritarian and patriarchal cultures as a correction of the disrespect and dominance doctors often show their patients.

CONCLUSION

Bioethics is now immersed in a multicultural world of medicine and science. It must appreciate the variety of values that surround health and healing in various cultures. It must introduce into its canon the philosophical discourse about moral relativism. Bioethics must be multicultural and, at the same time, ready to criticize practices that violate human dignity. The need for global comprehension of diverse moral values must be met by education. The challenge to another culture's moral values should be supported by skilled and articulate analysis of the grounds for such opposition.

BIBLIOGRAPHY

Alora, A., and J. Lumitao, eds. 2001. *Beyond a Western Bioethics: Voices from the Developing World.* Washington, DC: Georgetown University Press.

Fadiman, A. 1997. *The Spirit Catches You and You Fall Down: A Hmong Child, Her American Doctors and the Clash of Two Cultures.* New York: Farrar, Straus & Giroux.

Gupta, B. 2002. *Ethical Questions East and West.* Lanham, MD: Rowman & Littlefield.

Macklin, R. 1999. *Against Relativism: Cultural Diversity and the Search for Ethical Universals in Medicine.* New York: Oxford University Press.

Reich, W., ed. 1996. "Medical Ethics, History of," and "Medicine, Anthropology of," *Encyclopedia of Bioethics.* New York: Macmillan.

Rendtorff, J., and P. Kemp. 2000. *Basic Principles in European Bioethics and Biolaw*, 2 vols. Barcelona, Spain: Institute Borja for Bioethics.

Tao, J., ed. 2002. *Cross-Cultural Perspectives on the (Im)Possibility of Global Bioethics.* Dordrecht, Netherlands: Kluwer Academic Publishing.

TenHaave, H. 2001. *Bioethics in European Perspective.* Dordrecht, Netherlands: Kluwer Academic Publishing.

Tong, R., A. Donchin, and S. Dodds. 2005. *Feminist Bioethics, Human Rights, and the Developing World.* Lanham, MD: Rowman & Littlefield.

• *Topic 14* •

Animal Ethics

"Baboons Battered by Brain Researcher"

Animal protection committees (APCs) exist by law at all research institutions that use animals for research. These committees are required to have at least one public member. Imagine that you are a public member of the APC at a leading research institution. An investigator presents a protocol to study the neurological features of severe traumatic brain injury (the leading cause of death for children and young adults in the developed world—about two million people die each year from head trauma due to accidents, violence, or falls). He proposes to use baboons as experimental subjects. The animals would be sedated, placed in restraints, and subject to increasingly powerful blows to the head. The animals would be revived, then given a battery of behavioral tests and brain imaging. After a number of repetitions of this procedure, the animal would be euthanized and an autopsy done. One hundred animals would be used in these studies. How do you judge this protocol?

A colony of rhesus monkeys lives in a clean, well-designed facility. The monkeys are active, friendly, and seem to enjoy their life in captivity. However, at certain times, investigators take them to the laboratory where they are inoculated with human immunodeficiency virus (HIV). Rhesus monkeys are quite susceptible to this virus and contract most of the symptoms associated with AIDS. They are then treated with a variety of retroviral drugs to determine whether the drugs combat the virus. Other monkeys are vaccinated with experimental vaccines and then infected. Out of this research laboratory have come several AIDS drugs now in common use. The long search for an effective vaccine seems to be moving closer to achievement. This protocol comes up for annual review before your committee. How would you judge it?

The baboons and the monkeys in these stories are research animals. They serve science and human purposes at the cost of suffering and life. Their use is a bioethical issue.

Animals are omnipresent inhabitants of the biosphere. We humans are included in this vast population. However, in this topic, we will employ the word "animal" to refer to all nonhuman animals. This topic will examine the general question of the moral status of animals, then focus on one issue that connects the general question to biomedical ethics, namely, the use of animals in research.

Animals roam through human life in many ways. From ancient times, humans have hunted animals for food. Domestication of animals took place early in civilization. Animals provided transport and became weapons of war. Birds and animals of all sorts end their lives in abattoirs and finally on market counters. Multitudes of humans dwell with animal companions (often their only contact with animals in urban life). In addition, the changes made by humans in the physical world affect the lives of animals living in various environments. Turning prairie into farmland drives roaming ruminants away; cutting down forests wipes out populations of birds and animals adapted to forest life, pollutes streams, and drowns out fish life.

In recent years, the application of industrial techniques to raising animals for food has radically, and often cruelly, changed the natural life of chickens, pigs, and cattle. The relationship between humans and animals is, unquestionably, filled with ethical problems that have, in recent years, been much debated. The British Parliament has debated, almost yearly, the ethics of fox hunting in the English countryside and British law now prohibits the killing of foxes in the hunt; a California region famed for its restaurants was pressured to banish pâté de foie gras from menus because that delicacy comes from force-fed geese; dolphins at an aquatic park were liberated into the sea; minxes destined to become expensive fur coats have been freed from their farms. Many individuals and groups are dedicated to the welfare of animals. Some of them carry this dedication beyond debate to highly visible demonstrations.

The initial ethical question is, Why should any of this matter? For most of the history of Western civilization, humans have simply believed that animals existed for human use. In the opening chapter of the Hebrew Christian bible, the Lord says, "Let us make man in our image . . . and let them have dominion over the fishes of the sea and over the birds of the air, and over the cattle . . . and over all the earth" (Gen. 1:26). Buddhist and Hindu views, which believe that reincarnation cycles human and animal life and teach compassion toward all living things, put animals in a place of moral consideration that Western culture lacks. Even when the occasional Western philosopher reflects on the moral place of animals, it is to reinforce their utility for humans and to censure excessive cruelty, not so much for the sake of the dumb animals as for the rational humans who might develop habits of cruelty among themselves. Immanuel Kant wrote, "Animals are not self-conscious and are there merely as a means to an end. That end is man. . . . He who is cruel to animals becomes hard also in his dealings with men. . . . [T]ender feelings toward dumb animals develop humane feeling towards mankind."[1]

Nine years after Kant wrote those words, British philosopher Jeremy Bentham shifted the moral view about animals. He wrote, "The question is not, can they reason? Nor, can they talk? But, can they suffer?"[2] The past presumption that moral standing rested on rationality, the ability of beings to reason, discuss, agree, and contract with each other, was challenged. Bentham, who believed that the purpose of ethics was to prevent suffering and promote pleasure, encompassed the suffering and pleasures of all living beings in his "utilitarian calculus." His words came at a propitious time: in British society the keeping of pets had become fashionable, and a revulsion against cruel treatment of domestic animals urged the establishment of the Society for the Prevention of Cruelty to Animals (SPCA). Slowly, a reflective ethics about the place of animals in the human world and their treatment began to grow.

In its beginnings, that ethic combined the "human decency" concept enunciated by Kant and the sensitivity to suffering stated by Bentham. A strong utilitarian argument for humane treatment to animals could be made in a world where animals provided so much for human welfare and where losses of animals or deterioration in animal health could lead to human detriment. Cruelty to carriage and dray horses was an early cause of the SPCA. Even if one did not count the sum of animal suffering and pleasure in their overall welfare, the welfare of humans themselves depended in serious part on the welfare of their animal servants. Strangely enough, this view supported the conservation of animals for the hunt, considered an important masculine activity. The utilitarian argument also allowed an important loophole: certainly experimentation on animals for medical science contributed to human welfare and, thus, could be allowed, with due attention to prevention of unnecessary cruelty. Still, as philosopher Peter Singer of Princeton University famously pointed out in his book *Animal Liberation*, the interest of animals in not suffering and in pursuing their natural lives should be equal to the interests of other creatures: for humans simply and always to place their interests above animals is a sort of prejudice, a speciesism that has no basis in fact.

Some philosophers have argued that animals have rights—the right to be alive, to flourish in their natural setting, and to be free from humanly inflicted suffering. The ethical concept of rights is difficult enough to explain when applied to humans; it becomes quite problematic when applied to animals. In its historical meaning, *rights* seems to mean justifiable claims to be free from interference with one's life, property, and pursuits and, to some extent, claims to enjoy certain benefits within social life. Rights are often assumed to arise from some sort of social contract. In the world of animals, no such contract is possible, and the rational capacity that justifies these claims is not an animal characteristic. Still, some thinkers erase the boundaries between the rational possessors of rights and other beings that are simply "subjects of a life." Being alive with the characteristics of any species constitutes the ground for rights. Whatever the philosophical difficulties with the concept of rights, it forces humans to think about animals as beings in themselves, with spheres of influence, rather than simply as servants and subjects of human interests.

Also, *ethology*, the scientific study of animal behavior, has suggested many psychological and social similarities between animals and humans. Clearly, many animals appear to have emotions similar to humans; many species seem to exhibit traits usually considered moral in humans, such as cooperation, sympathy, and devotion to kin. The scientific findings of ethology frequently find their way into popular television shows about animals and become, in less scientific forms, common beliefs about the kinship between animals and humans.

This shift in moral focus has multiple implications: Should animals be confined or killed for food and clothing? Should hunting be allowed? Should animals be used in biomedical research? Should endangered species be protected at whatever cost to the human community? Should natural habitats be safeguarded and even improved for animal life? All of these questions inspire argument, and some arguments even lead to violence on the part of animal activists. Although Singer, one of the principal figures in bioethics, pioneered the general field of animal ethics, relatively few bioethicists have devoted careful attention to the issues. There is no mention of animals in Tom Beauchamp and James Childress's major treatise on bioethics. Barbara Orlans and colleagues have broken this relative silence with their book *The Human Use of Animals*, which explores the ethical aspects of almost every form of human-animal interaction, from training pets to medical research with animals. This latter issue is very close to bioethics since advances in the practice of human (and animal) medicine are, it is claimed, dependent on research using animals.

ANIMALS IN BIOMEDICAL EXPERIMENTATION

The use of animals became a standard feature of medical research during the nineteenth century: much of modern physiology originates in the vivisection and dissection of rats, dogs, and cats. Modern pharmacology tested drugs in animals. Until the latter half of the twentieth century, medical students learned the elements of surgery in the "dog lab." During the nineteenth century, powerful antivivisection movements appeared both in England and America. They exposed the terrible conditions and fate of laboratory animals and often claimed that little was accomplished for human health by this gratuitous suffering of animals. In Britain, the Cruelty to Animals Act of 1876 initiated a system of inspection and regulation of animal laboratories and required use of anesthesia for mutilating procedures. Not until 1966 did the United States regulate animal experimentation in ways that prohibited unnecessary suffering and prescribed humane living conditions for lab animals.

Over time, many alternatives to the use of animals were developed, and the dog lab almost disappeared from medical training (it is legally forbidden in Britain). Despite these reforms, many animal rights activists remain adamantly opposed to research with animals. They lobby legislatures and demonstrate at the National Institutes of Health. They break into research laboratories to steal records, destroy equipment, and liberate research animals. They sometimes harass researchers. They either deny that human benefit has resulted from research or declare that human benefits obtained by egregious violation of animal rights are ill-gotten gains.

As is often the case, moral polarities define the debate: animal activists repudiate any use of animals in research; researchers defend the use of animals as essential to scientific and medical progress. In practice, however, a middle ground maintains both that animals have moral status and also that human benefit sometimes justifies the use of animals. The philosophical basis of this middle ground rests on the proposition that animals do share with humans many of the central attributes that should inspire moral respect. At the same time, various species of animals possess these attributes in varying degrees. They enjoy a higher quality of life in relation to the extent and complexity of these attributes. Slugs, lizards, and fish do not inspire the moral respect that gorillas, dogs, and dolphins usually do. It is morally licit, in this view, to judge the permissibility of research in relationship to the nature of the animal and to balance the harms and the benefits of animal research against the human benefits that are expected.

Many animal advocates and researchers who occupy the moral middle ground have rallied around the "Three Rs," proposed by William Russell and Rex Burch in 1959: replacement, reduction, and refinement. Replacement requires that alternatives to the use of animals, such as computer simulation and cellular preparations, be used whenever possible. The safety of drugs, for example, can be tested in cloned human tissue rather than in animals. Reduction advises researchers to design experiments so as to minimize the numbers of animals used. Refinement demands that interventions be improved so as to reduce invasiveness and diminish pain.

In this view, ethical debates concern whether some sorts of experimentation are so damaging to the animal or to the species that they should be forbidden, whether alternatives can be found for certain studies, whether pain management is adequate, and whether the numbers and kinds of animals used can be restricted. These debates have resulted in extensive government regulation of animal research in most developed nations. In the United States, ethical review committees, or APCs, must approve of all federally funded research using animals. These committees oversee the living conditions and treatment of research animals and review protocols calling for animal use. A responsible review committee will assiduously hold researchers to the Three Rs. Still, it is undeniable that the utilitarian calculus of costs and benefits allocates most costs to the animals and most benefits to the humans (except, of course, in that portion of animal experimentation that aims to improve animal care and health).

The words of the founder of modern physiology, Claude Bernard, have faded into the past: "A physiologist . . . is absorbed by the scientific idea which he pursues: he no longer hears the cry of animals, he no longer sees the blood that flows, he sees only his idea and perceives only organisms concealing problems which he intends to solve."[3] Rather, most modern researchers would agree with the view of Bernard's contemporary, American philosopher William James, himself an experimental psychologist. James rejects the opinion that "it is no one's business what happens to an animal, so long as the individual who is handling it can plead that to increase science is his aim. . . . The rights of the helpless, even though they be brutes, must be protected by those who have superior power." He defended limits on animal research. The ethics of animal research now reflects the tension between an enhanced respect for animal life and the moral imperative to improve human life.[4]

NOTES

1. I. Kant, *Lectures on Ethics* (1780), trans. L. Infield (New York: Harper & Row, 1963), 239.

2. J. Bentham, *Principles of Morals and Legislation*, 1789, xvii, 1.

3. C. Bernard, *An Introduction to the Study of Experimental Medicine*, trans. T. Greene (New York: Henry Schuman, 1949), 103.

4. W. James, Letter, *New York Evening Post*, May 22, 1909.

BIBLIOGRAPHY

Cohen, C., and T. Regan. 2001. *The Animal Rights Debate.* Lanham, MD: Rowman & Littlefield.

DeGrazia, D. 1996. *Taking Animals Seriously. Mental Life and Moral Status.* Cambridge: Cambridge University Press.

Orlans, B., T. Beauchamp, R. Dresser, D. Morton, and J. Gluck. 1998. *The Human Use of Animals: Case Studies in Ethical Choice.* New York: Oxford University Press.

Regan, T. 1983. *The Case for Animal Rights.* Berkeley: University of California Press.

Regan, T., and P. Singer, eds. 1989. *Animal Rights and Human Obligations,* 2nd ed. Englewood Cliffs, NJ: Prentice Hall.

Reich, W., ed. 1995. "Animal Research," and "Animal Welfare and Rights," *The Encyclopedia of Bioethics.* New York: Macmillan.

Singer, P. 1990. *Animal Liberation,* 2nd ed. New York: Random House.

Smith, J., and K. Boyd. 1991. *Lives in the Balance: The Ethics of Using Animals in Research.* Oxford: Oxford University Press.

• *Topic 15* •

Environmental Ethics

"Farmers Oppose Genetically Engineered Crops"

$\mathscr{A}$pharmaceutical company has genetically engineered rice seed to contain a human protein that appears in tears and breast milk. That protein can be used to manufacture a medicine for diarrhea and anemia, two of the leading causes of the death of children under five in developing countries. The company seeks to plant their "pharm rice" in California's rice-rich Central Valley. Rice farmers oppose the project because they fear that the genetically engineered seeds could contaminate their own crops. Almost half of their crop is sold to Japan, where public concern supports very strict import restrictions on genetically engineered foods.[1]

Is this a story about bioethics or about environmental ethics? It is about human health: the health risks perceived by Japanese consumers are pitted against the possibility of medicine for children. It is about the environment: does genetically engineered seed contaminate crops? Certainly, many environmental issues affect human health, and decisions about how to deal with those issues involve ethical choices. Bioethics and environmental ethics touch at many points. However, environmental ethics is considered a subject quite distinct from bioethics. The terms *environment* or *environmental ethics* are not found in the indexes of bioethics books. Only one recent study, *The Ethics of*

This author is hardly expert in environmental ethics. He gratefully acknowledges help (and even some words) from Dr. Steven Kellert, Professor of Environmental Ethics at Yale University and two of Dr. Kellert's graduate students, Elizabeth Allison, Nicole Ardoin, and William Finnegan, colleagues of this author in an environmental ethics project. I am grateful for the help of one of the few bioethicists who is also an environmental ethicist, Professor Andy Jameton of the University of Nebraska.

167

Environmentally Responsible Health Care, links the concerns of environmental ethics and health care ethics by concentrating on the toxicity of health care practices.

We include the topic in this bioethics book for several reasons. First, the two fields do touch at many points and should communicate. Second, the Greek word *bios* means life in the widest sense; it does not refer just to the span of human existence between birth and death. Finally, as we mentioned in the introduction to part IV, we honor the man who invented the word "bioethics," Dr. Van Rensselaer Potter, who intended it to designate the study of human life within the encompassing and evolving life of the biosphere. While this brief chapter hardly achieves his goal, it acknowledges the unity between environmental ethics and bioethics.

"Environment" literally means "surroundings." When we say "environment," we obviously mean that it is we humans who are surrounded by all of these natural things. Yet, we ourselves are part of nature; our lives depend on the food that grows in the earth and the air we breath. Although we are constantly in contact with things that are man-made—our homes, clothing, cars, paved streets, school buildings and playing fields—we know that these man-made things are put together from the wood, metal, fibers, and fluids that come from nature. So, "environment" really means "us in our surroundings." We live in familiar environments and visit exotic ones. Everywhere, mountains, rivers, oceans, and forests surround the built world of cities. Yet, the physical world, omnipresent as it is, can almost become invisible to modern urbanites. The Victorian poet Gerard Manley Hopkins poignantly reflects the industrial Britain of his day:

> All is seared with trade; bleared and smeared with toil;
> And wears man's smudge and shares man's smell;
> The soil is bare now, nor can foot feel, being shod.[2]

Yet, when we look up to the mountains and out to the sea and through the forests, we call these things "nature." All those scenes of nature that seem so solid and real can be changed by human actions. Humans cut down forests, carve away mountains by mining, stop rivers with dams, spew noxious particles into air, and spill them into water. The exhalations of industry and autos warm the globe to the danger point. We are not only dependent on the natural world; we are changers, sometimes destroyers, of the natural world.

The ethical issues that appear as humans use and abuse their environment have become the subject of a special discipline, *environmental ethics*. The presence of human power in the natural world sets the problems for environmental ethics. It asks about the responsibilities of humans as they exert their powers to change the natural world and bend its resources to their needs. Environmental ethics is about how we humans should live in the natural world. Do we have duties toward nature? Could those duties ever require us to save some natural things, even if that means that we are inconvenienced or must make some sacrifice? What should we do to protect the natural world so that we and our descendants can continue to enjoy and benefit from it? How should we use the things of nature without using them up? Do the entities of the natural world—wild animals, trees, waterfalls—have a value in and of themselves that does not derive from any satisfaction, economic or aesthetic, that they might provide humans? Environmental ethics attempts to provide insight into these questions and to provide guidance about how to act upon those insights.

One standard theory of ethics, utilitarianism, offers a reasonable approach to this general problem of environmental ethics. Utilitarianism seeks to promote the greater good of the greater number of subjects. Without even delving into mysterious claims about the rights of animals and of trees and of minerals, utilitarian arguments can support the preservation of species and conservation of land and forests simply because their health and thriving are contributions to human welfare. Air pollution, for example, attacks human health; preservation of plants with potential medicinal properties contributes to human health. Actions that modify the environment have repercussions far into the future, as will our current production of the greenhouse gases that contribute to global warming. Future generations will be affected by our actions (or inactions) today, for many environmental effects are persistent and insidious.

Since human development of the land will certainly continue and increase, as human populations increase, a utilitarian argument would propose *sustainable development*, in which nothing more is taken out of nature than can be replaced by human effort and by nature itself. It was once thought that nature was inexhaustible: the seas would always be full of fish, the forests teeming with game, the earth always fertile, and clean water everywhere. It is now clear that human use exhausts natural resources. So-called renewable resources are so diminished that they cannot reproduce. Nonrenewable resources, such as coal, oil, and minerals, are simply used up.

Sustainable development is defined by the World Commission on Environment and Development (1987) as "development that meets the needs of the present without compromising the ability of future generations to meet their own needs." Sustainable development adds considerations of economic development to the notion of conservation. Sustainable development suggests that the lives of people around the world can be improved through the provision of nutritious food, clean drinking water, sanitation systems, modern health care and hygiene, affordable and accessible education, road networks, sturdy buildings, and reliable power sources; at the same time, we can protect and preserve natural environments and, in some cases, traditional cultures.

This concept raises complex questions that are as ethical as they are economic. How can resources be allocated equitably so that people in various countries get their "fair share"? Developed countries, particularly the United States, use a greater amount per capita of the world's natural resource: is this fair to people in poor countries? How do we account for the needs of future generations? How much of a supply of nonrenewable natural resources must we leave for them and for how long into the future? How much sacrifice should we demand from present generations in order to meet the needs of future generations? What quality of life should future generations inherit? These are questions with no clear solutions, but unless they are asked and answered, even unclearly and imperfectly, human life and the natural world will fail to support each other.

We have become familiar with conservation in daily life: recycling of cans, bottles, and paper is now common practice. Advice to limit use of water, electricity, and gas is frequently heard. Conservation often demands more stringent and often controversial strategies: limiting commercial fishing to protect stocks may seriously affect the livelihood of fisherman and the profitability of companies; limiting timber cutting has similar consequences. In particularly fragile ecosystems, such as wetlands and wildernesses, it may be necessary to exclude human intrusion so that the natural species can flourish: this is often a very controversial decision as the interminable debate over oil exploration in the Arctic Wildlife Refuge demonstrates.

The utilitarian approach is not, however, a simple one. In order to determine what constitutes a good, or the greater good of the greater number, complex calculations must be made. Costs must be calculated as well as benefits, and which effects will count as each must be determined. The beneficiaries of the good produced must be designated: the greater number may not be, as it superficially appears, the greater part of the population but, in some forms of utilitarian theory, those whose satisfaction would be greatest. Also, the lesser number in these calculations is left outside the distribution. Finally, there are problems peculiar to the environmental application of utilitarianism. That theory places satisfaction of conscious beings as its primary goal. Yet, it is not clear who, apart from humans and many higher animals, counts as conscious. Many more creatures, such as insects and plants, belong in the ecological community. Further, utilitarianism prizes utility, but many creatures in nature seem to offer no utility. A tiny owl that can only live in an old-growth forest and a lizard that can only survive in a sandy desert seem to bear little utility when compared with the cutting of trees for lumber or the development of housing. Calculation of utility, when the overall biosphere is the object of preservation, is enormously difficult.

Utilitarianism is a standard ethical theory. It works fairly well as a method of thinking about environmental problems. Yet, it may be that environmental ethics needs ethical concepts dissimilar to those of standard ethics since it (like animal ethics) engages with beings that cannot enter the rational deliberations, debates, and agreements so much a part of traditional ethics. The familiar ideas of mutual responsibilities, rights and duties, and respect for autonomy that fuel our ethical discourse must be reconfigured when nature, not other humans, is the other part of the ethical equation. The idea of community, built up of persons interacting, must be enlarged to include the interaction between humans and the natural world. The concept of justice also needs enlargement to fit into the wide natural world.

The concept of community is enlarged as we become familiar with ecological science. The modern science of ecology explains the relationship between organisms and their living and nonliving environments, revealing the interdependence of living things. Environmental scientists explore *ecosystems*, natural units of living and nonliving components that interact through chemical, material, and energy cycles to produce stable systems. The circular exchange of materials is the basic feature of an ecosystem. Within organisms, there are cycles of nitrogen, oxygen, and other elements that sustain organic life. Between organisms, predators absorb energy from prey in the food chain. At a global scale, the circulation of air masses and oceans affects climates, which in turn affect the cycles of life.

As the result of continuing adaptation to the diversity of conditions, an incredible number of species has developed over time. *Biodiversity* refers to the variety of life at all levels of biological organization, including the diversity within a species, between species, and among ecosystems. Ecosystems are interdependent. The stability of an ecosystem is the result of a complex web of interdependence and interaction. Food chains and nutrient cycles connect all elements of an ecosystem. Thus, damage to any one organism or characteristic of an ecosystem can affect the entire system. The Delhi Sands fly is a protected species. A large retail and residential project in southern California is being held up for its sake. This tiny creature is not so much loved for its own sake but for its role in an ecosystem. The fly is a pollinator of plants that live on neighboring sand dunes; the plants stabilize the dunes, and without the fly, the dunes will erode, changing the landscape. The fly is an essential player in that ecosystem.

The term *biosphere* is used to describe this vast interaction of energy. Human life exists within and as part of the biosphere. We depend upon the natural world for clean air, water, and food, among other needs. These cycles and material flows that support human life have been called *ecosystem services*. Yet, human population growth, industry, technology, and shortsighted development are responsible for destroying habitats, disrupting ecosystem services, and decreasing biological diversity. As a result, we humans are threatening our very life support system—the biosphere.

Moral philosophy has generally been blind to this view of humans as dwellers within the larger ecological community. Most moral philosophers (the ancient Stoics are the exception) have taken for granted that humans are integers, complete in themselves. These integers are sovereign beings, using the natural world for their own purposes and pleasures or, at most, struggling to overcome its strictures on human freedom. In contrast, environmental ethics draws on ecology to enlarge the concept of community. Humans are not independent of nature or sovereign to it but deeply embedded within it as a community of interest and justice.

Environmental justice also requires an enlargement of the notion of justice. The traditional notion concerns the distribution of benefits within a human social group. In any community, the benefits and burdens are distributed in various ways; some persons have more, and others have less. The question of justice arises when we ask whether any particular distribution of burdens and benefits is fair. Certain benefits, such as clean air and water, seem to be "common goods" that should be equally available to all persons in the community. Other distributions, such as personal wealth or political power, arise from differences in energy, effort, intelligence, and opportunity. Justice inquires whether those who possess such capabilities have a right to any greater share in social benefits.

In environmental ethics, the question of justice reaches further. It asks how human actions can maintain and restore harmony in nature. "A healthy ecosystem," say Jessica Pierce and Andrew Jameton, "is one that justifies—that is, balances or harmonizes—the complex relationships among its components."[3] Ecosystems are harmonious in themselves; even when one part destroys another, the destruction contributes to the support of the life of the system. Human behavior may disrupt those harmonies; thus, environmental justice seeks to restore them. It commands a certain reciprocity so that when something is taken from nature, something is returned. Seeking harmony, in which each part does what it should do and receives what it should receive, is a daunting challenge, particularly to economic and social systems built on the exploitation of nature for the good of a few.

The considerations reviewed here are, for the most part, *anthropocentric*; that is, they appreciate the natural world from our human viewpoint. It is a value for us. Many environmentalists prefer a *biocentric* view, which, in contrast to an anthropocentric view, sees nature as having value in itself, regardless of its human purposes. They argue that all living beings on the planet have the right to exist and that humans have the duty to ensure that habitats are healthy even for species that have no known human utility. One of the founders of environmental science, Aldo Leopold, wrote that "a thing is right when it tends to preserve the integrity, stability and beauty of the biotic community. It is wrong when it tends otherwise."[4] Ethical action, in any situation, would transcend the human-centered view and attempt to encompass the good of the biosphere. The animals, plants, and minerals that make it up and the cycles of energy that flow through it have intrinsic value, not just instrumental value for human use. Whatever has value in itself also has intrinsic rights to exist and to flourish.

The biologist Edward O. Wilson quotes a leading environmental ethicist, Holmes Rolston, in a passage that poses the deontological question, Do other species [than humans] have inalienable rights? Wilson writes, "[T]he philosopher Holmes Rolston III tells a story that can serve as a parable of this trend [toward biocentrism]. For many years at a subalpine campground in the Rocky Mountains he occasionally visited a sign that read, 'Please leave the flowers for others to enjoy.' When the wooden signs began to erode and flake, they were replaced by new ones that read, 'Let the flowers live!'"[5]

Environmental ethics has much work to do. Its first task is to show that human agency toward the physical world belongs in the realm of ethics. It must engender a deeper appreciation for the values of the natural world and a better understanding of the intricate connections between all its parts, including our human selves. This is best done by example, and there are multiple examples of this complexity, from the insect world to the atmosphere. Additionally, it must instill a sense of responsibility for human action and institutional behaviors that affect the biosphere. It must also analyze complex practical problems. Whenever we find that human action threatens the environment, human interests are involved both negatively and positively: negatively because human causes of environmental degradation bring disadvantages and disease to humans; positively because the causes themselves usually represent some human desire for improvement. Forests are cut because people need lumber to build homes or firewood for cooking. Mines are dug because the extracted minerals make the artifacts of our world. Coral reefs are threatened by the pollution coming from the resorts built to accommodate the tourists who come to enjoy them. At the heart of environmental ethics is the insistent question of how to respect the natural world and, at the same time, respect human life.

There are many points of contact between environmental health and human health. It has long been recognized that a degraded, polluted environment can cause disease: the Industrial Revolution in England brought widespread lung disease to "this other Eden, demi-paradise, this fortress built by Nature for herself against infection" (*Richard II*, I, 40). The public health movement began in England when it was recognized that polluted water sources generated cholera. It is now recognized that the clearing of forest habitats drives sources of infection into the human population. Modern science also now recognizes what native peoples have long known, that forests are sources of valuable botanical medications that may be lost when forests are devastated. Many environmental issues are relevant to bioethics. I shall, in conclusion, examine one of these.

GENETICALLY MODIFIED ORGANISMS

One practical problem in environmental ethics is closely linked to standard bioethics, although bioethicists have hardly participated in discussions about it. This is the problem of genetically modified organisms (GMOs) mentioned at the beginning of this topic. This issue connects with standard bioethics because it is an application of genetic science that has significant implications for human health. When geneticists learned to splice genes from one organism into another, they realized that they could do, rapidly and precisely, what farmers had done slowly for millennia. Farmers breed generation after generation of stock, using the stronger in each generation to propagate the next crop. Scientists can increase the productivity of crops by inserting into food plants genes that resist predators and disease. They can eliminate weeds without eliminating plants. They can stimulate milk production in cows.

Among these many achievements, one of the most remarkable is the genetic engineering of *Bacillus thuringiensis* (Bt), a bacterium that attacks the intestines of insects. Scientists cloned the genes that produce the toxin and inserted it into crop plants. The plant itself then produced the toxin, devastating the insects that preyed upon them. Corn, soybeans, potatoes, and many other crops now have the Bt gene and need not be sprayed with chemical pesticides. Also, their internal toxin attacks only the insects that attack them, not other innocuous creatures. Another remarkable achievement is "golden rice." A gene that produces beta-carotene, a precursor of vitamin A, has been integrated into rice that lacks that essential vitamin. Beta-carotene (which colors carrots yellow) makes up for vitamin A deficiency in vast populations dependant upon rice as their staple food.

These and many other scientific accomplishments are not unequivocal marvels. Even before these genetic techniques, the doctoring of farm animals with antibiotics for growth was implicated in human disease as resistant bacterial strains were transferred from animals to humans in food. There is a genuine bioethical problem here. GMOs have the potential to increase crop yield and nutrient values in a world where population is outgrowing agricultural resources. They also lessen dependence on agricultural methods that are environmentally destructive. At the same time, they are human interventions in the natural world, which can have negative effects unforeseeable at present. Contamination of other crops, the fear of the California rice farmers, is a persistent possibility. Long-term effects on human health are unknown and possibly unknowable for years to come. Certainly, all the known methods of testing for food safety can be applied to GMOs, but their novel nature may hide some noxious effects. Also, modified crops may escape and infect wild relatives, creating "superweeds." GMOs may have an effect on biodiversity, affecting insects that may have some beneficial role to play in the ecosystem.

These problems cast a shadow over GMOs. Agribusiness aggressively marketed GMOs, attempting to dominate and control farming. This prompted the suspicion that the desire for profit overwhelmed concern for safety. The effects of genetic modification were fearfully unknown. European countries, such as France and Germany, banned GMO crops and products. Prince Charles accused the producers of GMOs of "playing God." Research has been stifled; research crops have been vandalized.

The ethical arguments surrounding GMOs must not degenerate into ranting from opponents and slick propaganda from proponents. They must insistently focus on the most prudent, risk-avoiding strategies, based on the best available agricultural and genetic science. They must reveal the mercenary, unscrupulous practices of the food industry whenever it prefers profit to safety. They must consistently incorporate Leopold's principle of biotic balance, together with a principle of justice within the world community.

E. O. Wilson, one of America's leading environmentalists, summarizes the GMO debate: "The problem before us is how to feed billions of new mouths over the next several decades and save the rest of life at the same time, without being trapped in a Faustian bargain that threatens freedom and security. No one knows the exact solution to this dilemma."[6]

NOTES

1. "State's Rice Farmers Fear Biotech Incursion," *San Francisco Chronicle*, April 8, 2004, A1, A16.

2. G. M. Hopkins, "God's Grandeur," *Gerard Manley Hopkins: Selected Poems and Prose*, ed. W. Gardner (London: Penguin Books, 1953), 26

3. J. Pierce and A. Jameton, *The Ethics of Environmentally Responsible Health Care* (New York: Oxford University Press, 2003), 122.

4. A. Leopold, *A Sand County Almanac* (New York: Oxford University Press, 1949), 224.

5. E. Wilson, *The Future of Life* (New York: Knopf, 2002), 134.

6. Wilson, *Future of Life*, 118.

BIBLIOGRAPHY

Callicott, J. 1989. *In Defense of the Land Ethic: Essays in Environmental Philosophy.* Albany: State University of New York Press.

Hargrove, E. 1989. *Foundations of Environmental Ethics.* Englewood Cliffs, NJ: Prentice Hall.

Leopold, A. 1949. *A Sand County Almanac.* New York: Oxford University Press.

Nuffield Council on Bioethics. *Genetically Modified Crops: The Ethical and Social Issues,* at www.nuffieldbioethics.org.

Pence, G. 2001. *Designer Food: Mutant Harvest or Breadbasket of the World?* Lanham, MD: Rowman & Littlefield.

Pierce, J., and A. Jameton. 2003. *The Ethics of Environmentally Responsible Health Care.* New York: Oxford University Press.

Reich, W., ed. 1995. "Environmental Ethics," "Environmental Health and Disease," and "Hazardous Wastes and Toxic Substances," *Encyclopedia of Bioethics.* New York: Macmillan.

Rolston, H. 1988. *Environmental Ethics: Duties to and Values in the Natural World.* Philadelphia: Temple University Press.

Wilson, E. 2001. *The Future of Life.* New York: Knopf.

Conclusion

*Y*ears ago, a series of travelogue films that introduced people of the pre-travel world to exotic places always ended with the phrase, "And now we bid farewell to beautiful Bali," or wherever. So, now we bid farewell to bioethics. Beautiful it may not be, but interesting it is. I hope that this travelogue through the subject explains clearly what it is about, exhibits some of its landscape, and, perhaps, lures the reader to further exploration.

Yet, here at the end lingers a haunting doubt. Was it worth coming this far? Is bioethics really very important? Certainly, the questions raised in bioethics are important: they touch deeply the way we live and die and the ways science and society enhance or impair our image of ourselves and our ability to live humanely. Also, bioethicists boast about their voluminous writings, the frequent citations of their wise observations, and their role in the world of medical education and public policy. They can tell how their ideas have floated into laws and legal decisions and changed doctors' dealings with patients. Yet, we must admit, elegant bioethical arguments are often diluted by the time they reach these venues. Also, as is often the case in ethics, bioethicists' counsel may be more honored in the breach than in the observance. Many debates simply roll on, without resolution.

How important and useful, then, is bioethics? An odd intimation of its importance comes not from the numbers of books published, articles written, or quotes cited. It comes, ironically, from an accusation cast at bioethicists in recent years. Bioethicists see themselves as honest folk, respecting persons, beneficent, nonmaleficent, and just. Some critics see them as malefactors at worst, dupes at best.

Bioethicists who suggest reasonable arguments to justify abortion, stem cell research, or forgoing life-sustaining treatment have been branded as

177

collaborators in a "culture of death." Bioethicists who support brain criteria of death are the stooges of the transplant surgeons. Bioethicists who should criticize the dominance and greed of the medical and scientific establishment have become complacent colleagues and beneficiaries of that establishment. Bioethicists who contribute to debates over genetics are co-opted by the proponents of genetic medicine. Bioethicists who consult for pharmaceutical and biotech companies are seduced into becoming shills for these self-serving enterprises, putting ethical polish on the tarnished practices of these commercial ventures. Bioethicists are mired in hopeless conflicts of interest: they cannot uphold moral values and, at the same time, serve mammon. As one critic says, "[N]ext time you meet a bioethicists, pay close attention; he may look like a bioethicist, but when you peel back his mask, you just might see the ad-man smiling back."[1]

These aspersions on bioethics are, in an ironic way, signs of its importance. No one bothers with the conflicts of interest of uninfluential people. No one denounces the ideas of inarticulate, irrelevant speakers. If powerful institutions invite bioethicists in, they must have, or be seen to have, something to offer. As a practitioner of bioethics for thirty years, I repudiate these aspersions and consider them a distortion of the record. Still, there can be honest debate over the extent to which ethicists should participate in the work and with the institutions that they might be duty bound to criticize.

Some bioethicists may have become unwitting (or witting but avaricious) apologists for practices that deserve rebuke. Yet, the world of bioethics has become vigorous enough that those who stray will certainly be caught in the flurry of debate. The world of bioethics is, in fact, a world of continuing debate. Opinion must be defended by articulate argument. Anyone who adopts the title of bioethicist must enter that debate and defend his or her views. Perhaps this world of debate, beginning in academia and flowing into public discourse, is the most important contribution bioethics can make. This negative demonstration of the importance of bioethics may be an odd way to end this book. But it may also entice readers to look firsthand at the work of bioethicists and judge for themselves.

This bioethicist believes that bioethics is a decent attempt to lighten the load of the human predicament of which philosopher G. J. Warnock speaks. As we saw in part I, he suggests that our human predicament arises from the sad fact that we suffer from limited resources, limited information, limited intelligence, limited rationality, and limited sympathy. It is, he proposes, extremely difficult to satisfy human needs with these limited capacities. The questions of bioethics, Who lives? Who dies? Who decides? are certainly questions of great import. They must be approached with the enlarged intelligence and sympathy that Warnock believes ethical reflection can provide.

Cramped understanding and shriveled sympathy can distort those questions into dogmatic or prejudiced assertions and claims of infallibility and domination. Whenever life is in question, understanding, rationality, and sympathy should be plentiful. Bioethics is a deliberate attempt to open understanding and sympathy as we approach these great questions. And we all must approach them.

NOTE

1. Carl Elliot, "Not-So-Public Relations: How the Drug Industry Is Branding Itself with Bioethics," *Slate* (December 15, 2003).

BIBLIOGRAPHY

Evans, J. 2000. *Playing God? Human Genetic Engineering and the Rationalization of Public Bioethical Debate*. Chicago: University of Chicago Press.
Jonsen, A. 1998. *The Birth of Bioethics*. New York: Oxford University Press, chs. 10, 11.
Smith, W. 2000. *Culture of Death: The Assault on Medical Ethics in America*. San Francisco: Encounter Books.
Stevens, T. 2000. *Bioethics in America: Origins and Cultural Politics*. Baltimore: Johns Hopkins University Press.

· *Appendix A* ·

Précis of Moral Philosophy

$\mathscr{A}$ column titled "The Ethicist" appears in the *New York Times*. It is written by Randy Cohen, who is not trained in moral philosophy but is a person of sound common sense. He is also a regular guest on a radio show on which an interviewer introduced him with the words, "Randy Cohen, who meddles in the lives of our listeners. Randy, are you ready to meddle?" Cohen laughingly agreed. Persons who are trained in ethics might be offended by the assertion that they meddle in people's lives. Yet, the first renowned teacher of ethics in the Western cultural tradition, Socrates, was certainly a meddler. His motto, "the unexamined life is not worth living," announced his program. He incessantly questioned people about how they should live and act and, by his lancing logic, revealed that often they did not understand what they meant when they said such things as "a man should be courageous." Indeed, he showed that most people were very confused about their most definitive assertions. The Athenians dubbed him the "Gadfly of Athens." The stung citizens judged his insistent queries as meddling in the extreme and silenced him with a draught of poisonous hemlock.

Plato, who knew and revered Socrates, carried his questioning further and also created a positive vision that would guide questioners toward answers. He proposed that morality was a distinctive characteristic of the human soul, maintaining order and harmony between the different, often conflicting, functions of the soul: reason, desire, and emotion. That inner order of the soul arose from insight into the most fundamental truths about being, a knowledge attained only after serious discipline of mind and body. The value of morality was unique, not comparable with other sorts of human goods, such as pleasure, fame, power, or money. It is better to be wronged, he famously said, than to do wrong.

Aristotle, student of Plato, broadened the vision of ethics. He began by asking, What is the goal or purpose of life? Examining various answers to this question, he concluded that the purpose of life is happiness, not in the modern sense of enjoyment, but as the fulfillment of all powers of which humans are capable. Human powers are fulfilled when reason finds the right measure of emotion and desire and chooses in accord with that measure. Aristotle described the range of virtues that compose the ability to choose rightly. Justice and friendship are central moral virtues, but in the last analysis, the capacity to contemplate the truth of things constitutes the ultimate human virtue. The good man is completely integrated, of one mind with himself and with his friends.

Many ancient philosophers contributed to these reflections on the good life. The Epicureans maintained that the good life was pleasure alone, but a pleasure restrained by moderation lest it lead to destruction. The Stoics, perhaps the most influential of ancient philosophers, took a diametrically opposed position, teaching that pleasure and the desire for pleasure can mislead humans: they must learn to overcome emotion and subject it to reason. It is imperative that humans discern the path of reason by investigating the nature of self and the natural world: a natural law will guide the inquiring mind as it seeks self-preservation and perfection. The final great moralist of classical antiquity, the Roman statesman Marcus Tullius Cicero, wove Aristotelian and Platonic ideas about the nature of virtue together with the Stoic ideas of natural law and natural justice. Cicero, being a man of politics, took ethics further into the realm of action than his philosophical predecessors. He was concerned about how choices are made when values conflict. He sought the answer in the concept of justice: the basic moral rule is never to disadvantage another for one's own advantage. The basic purpose of this rule is to preserve peace in the social world.

These authors profoundly influenced the intellectual tradition of Western culture. In the cultures of the Eastern world, Buddhist and Confucian thought elaborated views about the purpose of life and the forms of behavior to achieve it. Those traditions, from very different premises, often arrive at advice not unlike the admonitions of the Western thinkers. In all these forms of ethical thought, the object is to design a picture of how persons should form their characters so as to pursue an ordered, effective, and collaborative life. Obviously, that picture is painted against a cultural background that makes each portrait distinctive, regardless of similarities. The Greek philosophers were speaking to wealthy, free citizens of small states built on slavery, in almost perpetual war with each other. The Stoic and Epicurean philosophers wrote for literate persons in a cosmopolitan culture with a highly structured political system. The description of virtues, such as wisdom, courage, and temperance, might share words and even definitions, but their realization in education and life was colored by the culture and the times.

Christianity added a new note into this ethical reflection. The Christian God, like the God of the Jews, creates the world and its human inhabitants and instructs them, by explicit commands, about how they should live. Ethics had to introduce ideas about commandments, principles, rules, and obligations that are rarely found in the ethical literature of antiquity. Although the Stoics spoke about morality in terms of "natural law" and Cicero ruminated about how persons faced with moral duties in conflict should choose the right course, the dominant interest of the ancients was the depiction of moral character. Also, the ancient philosophers provided no systematic sanctions for moral and immoral behavior.

The Christian fathers, who inherited the philosophical views of the pagan philosophers, also placed humans within an encompassing cosmos of eternal, natural, and civil law. Obedience to God's law won the reward of the heavenly vision of God; disobedience damned to eternal suffering in hell. Jewish scholars, who had long cherished this view of morality as law, did not, to the same extent, have to meld it with the philosophical ideas about human character inherited from pagan thought. Nor did they inspire obedience to the law of Yahweh by the fear of punishment but rather out of fidelity to the covenant that Yahweh makes with his chosen people.

For many centuries, then, in the West, ethics was discourse about the virtues appropriate for human life lived within the Christian vision and about the laws and rules that should govern behavior. Medieval theologians sought to explain how humans came to know these virtues and laws and how they were to sort out their obligations in varying states of life and in various situations of perplexity and conflict. These theologians were particularly intrigued by how human reason apprehended moral concepts and whether the human will was free in making choices. These reflections added a new dimension to ethics: beyond character and obligation, what were the roots of moral perception and judgment?

During the Enlightenment, this dimension became the almost exclusive interest of ethical reflection. The Scottish philosopher David Hume examined emotion as the root of moral judgment; the German philosopher Immanuel Kant placed moral judgment in human reason and banished self-interest, desire, and inclination from the grounds of morality. Ideas that had been elided began to be pulled apart. Earlier philosophers had acknowledged that acting out of the obligation imposed by moral law differed from acting to achieve some purpose or goal. Still, not until the Enlightenment did philosophers begin to see these distinct concepts as opposed. Kant insisted that duties flow from what he called the *categorical imperative*, respect for the moral law itself and not from the end accomplished. Hume, and later more explicitly, John Stuart Mill, claimed that the moral quality of an act came only from its *utility*, the end to which it was directed.

The utilitarian thesis, expounded by Mill, was that "actions are right in proportion as they tend to promote happiness, wrong as they tend to produce the reverse of happiness. . . . The standard is not the agent's own greatest happiness, but the greatest amount of happiness altogether," or in the words of Mill's mentor, Jeremy Bentham, "the greater good of the greater number."[1] For the next fifty years, moral philosophers scrutinized the moves of the utilitarian argument; rehearsing the strengths and weaknesses of utilitarian or consequentialist ethics was the métier of moral philosophers. Utilitarianism had to assault the massive construction of Kant's categorical imperative, and although Kant's argumentation had become less persuasive to modern moralists, the persistence of ethical imperatives that contradicted consequentialist reasoning had to be accounted for: was it really right, for example, to execute an innocent man to placate a destructive mob and keep the general peace?

The broad permission to subordinate individual good to a general good that utilitarianism seems to grant is limited by one interpretation of that theory. Many utilitarians are, to use the academic term, *rule utilitarians*; that is, they recognize that often the observance of certain rules will contribute to the pursuit of the general good. Certain rules can be considered absolute, in that, without them, human activities collapse into moral chaos. Thus, while a pure, or "act," utilitarian might say that one may tell the truth or a lie, depending on whether one or the other will effect the greater good, a rule utilitarian would assert that the rule against lying is necessary to maintain the common good of communication and trust.

In 1903, ethics took a new turn in the English-speaking world. British philosopher G. E. Moore published his book *Principia Ethica*. The title mimicked Isaac Newton's *Principia Mathematica* (1687), literally a "new beginning," in which he revolutionized thinking about motion and the cosmos with his demonstration of the law of universal gravitation. Moore equally intended to revolutionize ethics by his claim that "good" means a simple, unanalyzable, "nonnatural" property, and that all statements about what is good, or derivatively, about what is right, are not open to proof or disproof. Moore's very contentious proposal drew moral philosophers into a new path. They dwelt on what it means to use "moral words" rather than on what constitutes moral character and action.

By the mid-twentieth century, the idea that all ethical statements are equivalent to subjective assertions about what the speaker feels about the matter at hand was firmly entrenched. When someone says, "murder is wrong," he or she is saying nothing more than "I am repelled by murder"; or, as some critics of this doctrine put it, "Hitler is evil" simply means "I personally dislike Hitler." If this position is taken, moral argument becomes futile. Although fierce debate raged among moral philosophers over these issues (much more complex than this simple summary can convey), the problem was not so much that examining the meaning of moral terms was a frivolous activity; it was rather that moral philosophers had generally abandoned the ancient quest for an understanding of right and good action in order to rummage through a fascinating but futile question about the meaning of words. In the 1920s, a group of philosophers and scientists, called the Vienna Circle, and some of their English disciples at Cambridge University announced that ethical affirmations were nothing but expressions of personal emotion. This opinion spread throughout Anglo-American moral philosophy during the 1930s and 1940s. Moral philosophers, intrigued by these theoretical problems, engaged in *metaethics*, the logical analysis of the meaning of ethical terms.

Metaethics did not totally drown normative ethics, but it certainly discouraged interest in particular moral problems. Even those philosophers who remained interested in practical ethics worked at a rather speculative level. They had to work under the constant shadow of metaethical critique and, thus, had to be cautious about the "truth value" of any affirmation. They remained on the relatively safe ground of *normative theory*, that is, the description of the structure of ethical arguments. Cambridge philosopher, C. D. Broad, suggested that all forms of argument about obligation could be distinguished into *deontological* and *teleological*, or *consequentialist*, forms. By midcentury, this distinction became canonical in normative ethics. The first form of ethical reasoning came to be called deontological from the Greek word for "duty." It was Kantian in inspiration and stressed obligation based on rules. The second form was called teleological, or more commonly, consequentialist. It was utilitarian in form, under Mill's inspiration. Although ethical theory is much more elaborate than these two types suggest, it is common to find ethics books announcing that there are two types of ethical theory, deontological and consequentialist, and that ethical problems must be resolved by having recourse exclusively to one or the other. Moral philosophers roamed through these constructions of reason and strayed far from moral experience.

Some moral philosophers were aroused from their "dogmatic slumber," as Kant said Hume's ideas had awakened him, by the public events of the American 1960s. The civil rights movement swept through the nation. Moral claims to equality among the races and redress of terrible injustices were demanded in massive demonstrations. The doubts of citizens about the wisdom and the rightness of the war in Southeast Asia grew into storm clouds of public protest that pushed a president from office. Both civil rights and war protests, while profoundly political, drew on deep moral convictions; intense moral conversations engaged citizens everywhere but nowhere more vigorously than in the universities. Professors of philosophy were lured out of the ivory tower into the maelstrom of debate. Many realized that their discipline did not take them very far on the path toward public moral discourse. In 1971, a cadre of leading philosophers founded a new journal, *Philosophy and Public Affairs*, in which they attempted to engage the practical dilemmas of moral experience. Some of the earliest bioethical essays appeared in that journal. Bioethics was one of the fruits of this new interest in practical ethics. In a sense, philosophers were rediscovering the vocation that Socrates, the first ethicist, had followed, urging people to live an examined life.

It is sometimes said, despairingly or disparagingly, that philosophy asks more questions than it answers. Certainly Socrates did that and frustrated his fellow citizens to the point of silencing him by execution. Today, a discipline that asks too many questions is more likely to provoke boredom than anger. We ask questions because we need answers to run our businesses, settle our finances, elect our leaders, and pass our laws. However, the philosophical questions that always seem to pop up, even after a seemingly good answer has been given, serve a different purpose. They lead the inquiring mind further, opening up a broader view of the problem. They stake out the uncertainties of which we must be aware as we move forward. They shake the certitudes that often lead to discrimination, domination, fanaticism, and destruction. A philosophical question is not merely an admission of ignorance; it is an invitation to reflection. So, in ethics, and in bioethics, many questions have been well answered, but all answers are open to new questions.

As this appendix closes, it might be worthwhile to reflect briefly on a very large question: what is morality all about? Even a superficial review of the vast literature of ethics reveals many different answers to that question. Regardless of the variety of scholarly answers, it is indubitable that human beings, in every culture and era that we know, affirm that some forms of action are right and others wrong. They all hold up certain sorts of persons as admirable and others as despicable. They praise and blame, counsel and command, reward and punish. Certainly, they do all these things rather differently and invoke different standards so that it is sometimes hard to find common ground. Still, the fact of morality is apparent. Less common but still widespread is the deliberate effort to articulate the reasons behind this universal fact. Some cultures, Hindu and Buddhist, for example, are permeated with a rich moral vision; others acknowledge a more codified yet deep formulation of duties and virtues, as in Confucian, Christian, Jewish, and Islamic societies. In part I, we offered Prof. G. J. Warnock's view that ethics is about the amelioration of the human predicament. This is, I think, a good characterization, but it is far from definitive. If there were a definitive answer, the voices of philosophers, priests, poets, and parents "ethicizing" through the centuries would fall into silence.

It should be clear now why ethicists might resent being called "meddlers in people's lives." Those who come from the intellectual tradition of ethics believe that they are equipped by their education to help with the definition of ethical words, to outline the features of ethical issues, and to suggest how arguments might be evaluated, but never to tell anyone what to do. On the other hand, they certainly are surreptitious meddlers. They would prefer that people saw things as clearly as they believe they do. They are, while remaining reticent about what is right and wrong, convinced that people would be more likely to do rightly if they better understood a given problem and reflected on it, as the great philosopher David Hume once said, "in a calm, cool moment."

NOTE

1. J. S. Mill, *Utilitarianism*, ch. 2; J. Bentham, *Principles of Morals and Legislation*, I, 13.

BIBLIOGRAPHY

Becker, L., and C. Becker, eds. 2001. *Encyclopedia of Ethics*. New York: Routledge.
Blackburn, S. 2000. *Being Good*. New York: Oxford University Press.
Frankena, W. K. 1973. *Ethics*. Englewood Cliffs, NJ: Prentice Hall.
Gibbard, A. 1990. *Wise Choices, Apt Feelings: A Theory of Normative Judgment*. Cambridge, MA: Harvard University Press.
Hampshire, S. 1983. *Morality and Conflict*. Cambridge, MA: Harvard University Press.
Hare, R. M. 1981. *Moral Thinking: Its Levels, Method, and Point*. Oxford: Clarendon Press.
MacIntyre, A. 1978. *A Short History of Ethics: A History of Moral Philosophy from the Homeric Age to the Twentieth Century*. New York: Macmillan.
Timmons, M. 2002. *Moral Theory. An Introduction*. Lanham, MD: Rowman & Littlefield.
Warnock, G. J. 1971. *The Object of Morality*. London: Methuen and Company.

• *Appendix B* •

Précis of the History of Medical Ethics

$\mathcal{M}$edicine is the attempt by one person to heal the wounds or illness of another by using special skills and talents. It is a most ancient and ubiquitous human practice. It takes many forms, from prayer and enchantment to drugs and surgery. Whatever its form, it brings two persons into an especially intimate relationship, where trust must accompany skill. The general concept of medical ethics deals with the ways in which that relationship is understood. Certain responsibilities and duties, limitations and restraints guide behavior in that relationship.

Western scientific medicine names that long history of healing that relies on careful observation of the origin and progress of disease, the discovery of causes and influences, and the application of physical means, such as drugs and surgery. Medicine of this sort is primarily working with nature and the body rather than with the supernatural and the spirit. The history of this form of medicine begins in the fifth century and is associated with the school of Hippocrates. Hippocrates was a historical figure, but his "school" was not a locus of learning in which he was professor with a class of medical students (although it is associated in legend with a temple of healing on the Greek island of Cos). Rather, the school consists of a collection of writings from many authors over a several-century period. The historical Hippocrates may have written some of these treatises, but the entire collection bore his name, reflecting the great prestige in which he was held.

The collection contains descriptions of disease and treatments. It also contains a few treatises on the behavior of doctors in relation to their patients. However, in one of the medical texts, a single sentence epitomizes the ethic of the Hippocratic physician. It says simply, "with regard to diseases, note two things: be of benefit and do no harm" (*Epidemics* I, xi). In general, the Hippocratic ethic requires the physician to care assiduously for his patients, to treat them with courtesy, to dispense with fees for those who cannot pay, and to refrain from telling them anything that would frighten them. The most explicit statement of the Hippocratic ethic comes in a document called *The Oath*, probably written several centuries after the life of Hippocrates. *The Oath* appears to be a solemn affirmation of the physician's duties, taken at the moment of admission into some sort of medical guild or society, possibly associated with an ancient religious sect.

After an invocation of the gods of healing, *The Oath* begins with a statement of gratitude and fidelity to one's teachers. It then affirms, in words similar to the injunction above, "I will use treatment to help the sick according to my ability and judgment and never to bring them harm or injustice." A few lines further on, the injunction is echoed, "[I]nto whatever houses I enter, I will enter to help the sick, and I will abstain from all intentional injustice and harm." This phrase becomes more specific, explicitly mentioning the harm of sexual exploitation "of man or woman, bond or free." *The Oath* enjoins the giving of poisons to cause death, even if requested. It forbids assisting in an abortion. It requires the physician to keep confidential whatever he learns about his patients. Although historians interpret these injunctions variously, they have passed into the traditional ethics of Western medicine.

As Christianity became the dominant faith of Europe, its moral teaching infiltrated medical ethics. Christianity inherited from Judaism a powerful belief in the sovereignty of God over all life and death. The sanctity of life is a central moral tenet of both faiths. The prohibition of killing and abortion, found in the Greek *Oath*, is reinforced by Church teaching that they are sinful. However, one feature of Christian morality becomes particularly salient: the obligation of care for the poor. Barely mentioned in the Hippocratic texts, this duty is constantly invoked in Christian teaching about medicine. Church teachers often cite a passage from the Gospel of St. Luke in which a Samaritan "has compassion upon" a wounded Jew, his enemy, treats his wounds, and pays for his care at a hostelry (Luke 10: 25–37). Compassion and charitable care become central features of medical ethics.

In the early Christian centuries, monks practiced medicine and were forbidden to request payment. As medicine became a lay activity in the Middle Ages, physicians were reminded that they had a moral obligation to serve the poor. The church supported hospitals in which the poor were cared for. Religious orders dedicated themselves to this work. The Brethren of the Hospital of St. John of Jerusalem (later known as the Knights of Malta) followed a rule that commanded service "to our lords the sick." Fulfilling the duty of charity and making a living from medicine posed a moral dilemma for lay physicians. One medieval physician recommended a solution to the dilemma: "You must treat the poor for the love of God; you can make the rich pay dearly!"

During the late Middle Ages, medicine became a scholarly subject taught in universities. A medical profession, primarily of learned doctors, began to form throughout Europe, although most healers were self-taught or tutored. Physicians founded medical guilds that served the profession by setting conditions and controls on who could practice and how much could be charged and also maintained the tradition of charitable care. As the profession emerged, new rules governing the relationship between practitioners were formulated. In the Renaissance, the rediscovery of the Hippocratic literature revived interest in ancient medicine. Medical competence was seen not merely as possession of a lore and some physical skills: it was also a mastery of the "science" of medicine, elaborated in the ancient texts. Also, the ethical tenets of *The Oath* and other Hippocratic writings were the subject of scholarly commentary. After a long lapse, *The Oath* became the epitome of medical ethics.

By the end of the eighteenth century, an elaborate ethical code had developed around the fundamental imperatives of benefit to patients and compassion for the sick. Physicians must attain competence, maintain confidentiality about their patients, care for those who cannot afford to pay, and never abuse the trust of their patients, particularly by enticing them into sexual relations. This ethic, certainly often breached by greedy and ignorant doctors, was nevertheless constantly proclaimed. In 1802, a British physician, Thomas Percival, wrote the first book entitled *Medical Ethics*. He formulated his ethics into a set of seventy-two precepts, forming a "code." He advised sympathy and patience with patients, sensitivity in communication, and confidentiality, courtesy, firm discretion, and respect for precedence in dealing with colleagues and consultants. Physicians must, he wrote, "unite tenderness with steadiness, and condescension with authority, so as to inspire the mind of their patients with gratitude, respect and confidence."[1] Percival's book was widely praised. In 1847, the newly established American Medical Association adapted it to serve as its Code of Medical Ethics. Although medical ethics might be interpreted as advertising for the profession rather than physicians' sincere intention to serve their patients, the rules did serve to protect patients against rapacious, careless, and deceitful practitioners.

In the mid-twentieth century, this long tradition was challenged. Medical science was creating new technological solutions, making medicine much more effective than ever before. The pharmaceutical technologies, particularly antibiotics, repelled lethal diseases. Other technologies supported life by mechanical means. They were able to substitute for impaired breathing, for irregular heartbeat, for damaged kidneys, for imbalanced metabolism, and for missing enzymes and vitamins. Often their effectiveness seemed limited to changes in physiological status, with little improvement in the quality of the patient's life. Rapid innovations in the use of powerful drugs to treat cancer seemed to extend life but often not for long, and the life that was sustained was often marred by the toxic effect of the drugs. Patients whose cancer disappeared for a time, often relapsed and, after another bout of chemotherapy, died. The ventilator, invented to support breathing compromised by acute respiratory crisis, now was used to support life when hope of recovery was lost, even for patients who had permanently lost consciousness. Almost every medical miracle, undoubtedly beneficial for many, could be harmful to others, even to those who benefited. So, in the early 1960s, remarkable medical achievements posed the moral conundrum of modern medicine. The ancient maxim of Hippocrates was "be of benefit and do no harm." Now questions had to be added to that maxim: What is benefit and what is harm? Who should enjoy the benefit and who must go without? So, the questions asked in the opening chapter of this book, Who lives? Who dies? Who decides? became the themes of the new ethics of medicine, called bioethics.

NOTE

1. T. Percival, *Medical Ethics*, ed. C. Leake (Baltimore: Williams and Wilkins, 1927), 1, 71.

BIBLIOGRAPHY

Jonsen, A. 2000. *A Short History of Medical Ethics*. New York: Oxford University Press.
Miles, S. 2004. *The Hippocratic Oath and the Ethics of Medicine*. New York: Oxford University Press.

· Appendix C ·

The Frankenstein Analogy

$\mathscr{I}$t is not uncommon to find reference to Frankenstein in bioethical writings, particularly in the popular media. An implantable artificial heart reminds some author of the Frankenstein story. Transplantation of organs recalls the grisly creation of Frankenstein's monster out of parts snatched from cadavers. Genetically engineered organisms and plants are called "Frankenbugs" and "Frankenfood." It is interesting to examine the relevance of this simile for the issues of bioethics.

The story of Frankenstein was written in an era when science was on the verge of the developments that make bioethics necessary. In the early eighteenth century, brilliant minds examined the mysterious workings of the human body with new interest and ingenuity. Chemistry, which for a century had dissolved minerals and analyzed fluids, began to turn to the composition of the human organism. In the early nineteenth century, the students of "animal chemistry" studied the processes of digestion and described the components of food even as we still do, as *oleaginous* (fats), *saccharinous* (carbohydrates), and *albuminous* (proteins). The field of physiological chemistry was born and, for the rest of the nineteenth century, unraveled the ways in which life is originated and sustained by respiration, nutrition, and elimination. Oxygen became a topic of avid study. Cellular theory and germ theory revolutionized the understanding of disease. The structure of tissues and the hitherto hidden marvels of reproduction were observed through the microscope.

Also at the end of the eighteenth century, physics, which had lived in the glory of Newton's laws of motion and theory of gravity, began to investigate the physics of life. Electricity seemed to link nonliving and living matter. The nature of electrical charges was described in the 1780s. In 1792, Italian anatomist Luigi Galvani (rather, his wife) noted that the muscles of severed

193

frog legs contracted and twitched when stimulated with an electric shock. The term *galvanism* was coined to describe the power of electromagnetic force (imagined as a sort of fluid) to animate organic matter. In the same year, Alessandro Volta published studies on the electrical stimulation of muscles and several years later invented the battery to generate electrical power.

THE FRANKENSTEIN ANALOGY

While chemists and physicists worked in their laboratories, a literary party vacationed at a lake near Geneva. Two of England's most famous poets, George Gordon Lord Byron and Percy Bysshe Shelley, rented adjoining villas. With Shelley was his lover and future wife, Mary Wollstonecraft Godwin (she was nineteen years old). They passed stormy evenings telling ghost stories. One night, June 15, 1816, to be exact, Byron, Shelley, and another guest, Dr. John Polidori, discussed "the principle of life." In the language of the time, "principle" meant origin, source, first cause. For example, John Hunter, greatest English physician of the time, considered blood the "life-principle," distinguishing the living from nonliving. Shelley and Polidori were both interested in scientific investigation and were familiar with the work of the esteemed scientist and physician Dr. Erasmus Darwin (Charles Darwin's grandfather), who had investigated galvanism. During that evening conversation, the poets had speculated that "perhaps a corpse would be reanimated; galvanism had given token of such things; perhaps the component parts of a creature might be manufactured, brought together, and endued with vital warmth." Mary, "a devout but nearly silent listener" to that fascinating conversation, recorded those words. She could not sleep that night but saw "with acute mental vision" the shaping of a story. During that sleepless night, her imagination gave birth to her novel *Frankenstein*. That famous book could be called the first text for bioethics.[1]

The story is well known. Victor Frankenstein is a brilliant student of science, particularly of chemistry and physiology. While still at university, he is entranced by the idea of creating a living creature by means of galvanism. His motives are noble: "wealth was an inferior object; but what glory would attend the discovery if I could banish disease from the human frame and render man invulnerable to any but a violent death." His intense studies finally shed on his mind "a light so brilliant and wondrous . . . the astonishing secret . . . the cause of generation and life, nay more, I became myself capable of bestowing animation upon lifeless matter." He decides to compose a creature "like himself . . . and give life to an animal as complex and wonderful as man." He collects and composes all the needed parts from cadavers, then jolts the stitched amalgam with an electric shock from a "powerful machine." The composite cadaver comes to life. Frankenstein, however, is horrified by his creation and repudiates it. The "monster" or "wretch," as Frankenstein calls it, desperately seeks to understand how he came into being and to express his feelings in language. He yearns for acceptance by humans. He masters language but wanders alone, never welcomed into the human community. Rejection turns his originally benevolent nature to bitterness and violence. He tells Frankenstein, "I was benevolent and good; misery made me a fiend. Make me happy and I shall again be virtuous." His creator cannot make him happy, and in the end, the monster, now called the "fiend," kills its creator. In 1931, a film, starring Boris Karloff, vividly, though rather inaccurately, visualizes the novel. It is still a staple of late night movies.

Mary Shelley's novel was more than a chilling ghost story. It was a moralizing tale. She subtitled it, "The Modern Prometheus." Her readers, familiar with classical legend and literature, would have immediately understood. Those who recognize the reference today recall that Prometheus was a rebel Titan who stole fire from the gods and brought it to mankind, a theft for which he was grievously punished. However, the classically trained reader would also recall Prometheus Plasticator, Prometheus the Maker, who shaped the human form from clay, readying it to receive heavenly fire as the cause of its life and thought. Ancient literature portrays this artist as less than competent and relates that many human ills result from his less than perfect job.

Victor Frankenstein is a modern Prometheus, hoping to create a beautiful being of great power and ingenuity but failing. The monster blames his creator for his unhappiness and for his crimes. Mary Shelley wrote a warning for those who would carry their science into the mysteries of the creation of life. To affirm that this fantastic story was not mere imagination, Mary's husband, Percy, opened the preface that he composed for the first edition with the words, "The event on which this fiction is founded, has been supposed, by Dr. Darwin, and some of the physiological writers of German, as not of impossible occurrence." This was a moral tale about science and its future achievements.

I said that *Frankenstein* could be considered the first text of bioethics. That claim is rather melodramatic and needs some clarification. First, I do not mean that modern medicine and biological science is a horror story, telling how scientists create, willy-nilly, monsters rather than miracles. Bioethics is not a rounding condemnation of medical science (although some would make it so). It is not even a detective story, trying to find evil machinations behind each miracle. For while science can go wrong and medicine can harm instead of healing, their general direction has been toward human benefit. It is a kind of moralistic paranoia that wants to suspect evil in every good. Still, the story of Victor Frankenstein contains some of the essential elements of modern bioethics. First, it is a story about life. The "bio" in bioethics means "life." The word "life" is itself ambiguous. It can mean the course of a person's history from birth to death. Its major moments can be listed in a "bio" or picturesquely or poignantly described in a biography. It can also mean the processes that sustain organic life, the complex activities of cells, programmed by genes, in interaction with a nourishing environment. All of the "bio" sciences—biology, biochemistry, biophysics—study facets of these processes.

The fictional Frankenstein immerses himself in these studies (in their very immature forms) and burns to bring them from theory to practice. He succeeds in creating life in a cadaver; he has found the principle of life. He wants to "banish disease from the human frame." His scientific quest has a healing goal; it is meant to provide ultimate success to the medical task, which is, in Hippocrates's words, "to alleviate pain and lessen the violence of disease" (*The Art*, iii). Medicine deals with life in the biological sense and equally with life in the biographical sense. Physicians manipulate biological processes so that the life course of an individual can go on without pain or disability. They must know the biographies of their patients as well as their biology. In dealing with the patient as a person, physicians must observe standards of behavior that we call "ethics," the other half of the word bioethics. Even more, the power of science must be ethically employed as it is brought into contact with human life. So, the Frankenstein story, in which a scientist revives a living being and then must decide how to behave in relation to it, is an anticipation of bioethics.

Modern bioscience has yet to restore life after death has fully taken place. However, it can initiate life, imitating sexual reproduction in a laboratory dish, and it can sustain life as a merely organic process after personal life has disappeared. It cannot compose a complete human being out of exhumed organs and impart life to it. However, it can lift organs from a cadaver and implant them in a person whose own organs have failed. It can substitute mechanical devices for organic parts and functions. Whenever it performs one of these actions, it encounters the standards of behavior we call ethics because the action is performed not in a chemical preparation or physical device but with a human person. The work of bioethics is to examine the points at which the biosciences touch human life in individuals and in societies. The purpose of the examination is to discern how the science and its products can bring benefits with as little harm as possible. Bioethics seeks to form a picture of human persons and human society that can guide the vision and intentions of scientists.

Mary Shelly bestowed on Victor Frankenstein the title the Modern Prometheus because he sought to do what the legendary Titan did, namely, to make a human being. The modern biosciences all conspire toward the same goal. The modern making of humans consists in the correction of the physical and mental faults and failures that bring disease and death. Making is an activity in which the mind forms an image of something that will come into being as the hands manipulate material to match that image. Human purposes and motives guide the making and decide what is to be done with the product.

NOTE

1. M. W. Shelley, *Frankenstein* (London: Penguin Books, 1992), 8, 39–40, 51, 97, 11, 40.

BIBLIOGRAPHY

Hindle, M. 1994. *Mary Shelley's Frankenstein*. Penguin Critical Study. London: Penguin Books.
Shelley, M. 1992. *Frankenstein*. London: Penguin Books.

Glossary

autonomy   the moral status of being independent and self-directing by deliberated choice.

beneficence   the moral rule that directs persons to act in ways that benefit other individuals or society.

bioethics   "the systematic study of the moral dimensions—including moral vision, decisions, conduct and policies—of the life sciences and health care, employing a variety of ethical methodologies in an interdisciplinary setting" (*Encyclopedia of Bioethics*, "bioethics").

casuistry   a moral theory that aims to resolve individual ethical dilemmas by studying the circumstances of the case.

consequentialism   see teleology.

deontology   a moral theory that locates the foundations of moral judgments in principles and rules (also called formalism).

ethics   "the philosophical study of morality. . . . Its principal substantive questions are what ends we ought, as fully rational beings, to choose and pursue and what moral principles should govern our choices and pursuits" (*Cambridge Dictionary of Philosophy*, 284).

justice   the moral theory that deals with the fair and equal distribution of burdens and benefits within a community.

morality   "an informal public system applying to all rational persons, governing behavior that affects others, having the lessening of evil or harm as its goal, and including what are commonly known as the moral rules, moral ideals, and moral virtues" (*Cambridge Dictionary of Philosophy*, 586).

nonmaleficence   the moral rule that directs persons not to cause harm to others or to society.

paternalism   a judgment made for the benefit of another person, contrary to that person's own wishes, by a person who has or assumes authority. Soft, or justifiable, paternalism takes place when the person for whom the judgment is made is incapable of judgment, due to immaturity or temporary debility.

respect for autonomy   the moral principle that requires persons to refrain from preventing or interfering with the intentions, choices, and actions of others, unless those choices and actions inhibit the choices of third parties.

teleology   a moral theory that locates the foundation of moral judgments in the effects that follow from, or are intended to follow from, rational choices (also called consequentialism).

utilitarianism   a moral theory, a form of moral teleology, that states as the most basic principle of morality that human actions should aim toward the greater good of the greater number of persons.

After Part II

abortion   the termination of a pregnancy, either spontaneously or deliberately, by pharmacological or surgical intervention.

advance directive   a document stating that the signatory does not wish to have life-sustaining procedures in the event of terminal illness. These documents have legal validity in most American states.

assisted reproduction   a number of medical procedures intended to aid couples who are unable to procreate, due to physical defects in either partner; most commonly the procedures consist of artificial insemination with sperm from spouse or donor and in vitro fertilization and embryo transfer.

assisted suicide   voluntary euthanasia by a competent, terminally ill person with the aid of a physician, who provides and/or administers a lethal substance.

blastocyst   a preimplantation embryo of thirty to one hundred fifty cells. The blastocyst consists of a sphere made up of an outer layer of cells, a fluid-filled cavity, and a cluster of cells on the interior.

death, uniform definition of   irreversible cessation of circulatory and respiratory functions or irreversible cessation of all functions of the entire brain, including the brain stem.

durable power of attorney   a legal device whereby a person transfers the authority to make decisions regarding medical care to another trusted party, to be effective after the loss of mental capacity.

embryo   the immediate product of fertilization of sperm and ovum, in humans, from fertilization until the end of the eighth week of gestation. The earliest forms of embryonic life are called *zygote* (up to fifth day) and *blastocyst* (from sixth day to implantation).

euthanasia "good death," that is, the deliberate ending of life for the good of the person whose life is ended. Euthanasia may be voluntary, that is, done at the request of the patient, or nonvoluntary if the patient is incompetent to make the request. It may be performed by withdrawing or withholding life support (sometimes called *passive euthanasia*) or by direct administration of lethal substances (sometimes called *active euthanasia*). Euthanasia is illegal everywhere except in the Netherlands, Belgium, Switzerland, and in the United States in the state of Oregon.

fetus the developing product of the fertilization of an ovum in a female uterus, after the embryonic stage (in humans, eight weeks after fertilization) up to delivery.

gamete a male or female reproductive cell; sperm and ovum.

in vitro fertilization joining sperm and ovum outside the body of a woman, in a laboratory dish, to create an embryo. The resulting embryo can be implanted in a woman's reproductive organs to develop into a fetus or frozen for storage and future implantation.

informed consent the willing and comprehending acceptance of medical treatment, after being provided with appropriate information about the nature of the condition, the risks and benefits of treatment or nontreatment, and the recommendation of the physician.

organ donation a deliberate choice by a person to allow vital organs to be taken from his or her body for transplantation into another. The donation may be made by a living donor, unless the organ is essential to life, when it is made after declaration of death.

preimplantation genetic diagnosis (PGD) the search for a genetic mutation in a single cell taken from a four-cell embryo created in vitro.

primitive streak an initial band of cells appearing about fourteen days after fertilization, from which embryonic structures begin to develop. The primitive streak establishes and reveals the embryo's head and tail and left-right orientation and marks the beginning of organ development.

surrogate decision maker a person designated by law or by instruction of a person to make decisions on that person's behalf if they should become mentally incapacitated.

surrogate mother a woman in whose womb an embryo, created from the ovum of another woman, is implanted to be carried to term.

vegetative state a neurological condition in which serious damage to the brain deprives a person of the capacity for conscious and purposeful interaction with the environment, while leaving intact the capacity for breathing, reflex actions, and other vegetative functions. This state is called persistent vegetative state (PVS) if there is no recovery after three months following anoxic injury or one year after traumatic injury.

After Part III

adult stem cell   An undifferentiated cell found in a differentiated tissue that can renew itself and (with certain limitations) differentiate to yield all the specialized cell types of the tissue from which it originated.

amniocentesis   the technique of inserting a fine needle into the pregnant uterus and withdrawing a sample of amniotic fluid containing fetal cells that can be analyzed for genetic defects.

cerebral cortex   a layer of neuronal cells covering the cerebrum, controlling and integrating voluntary movement, vision, hearing, tactile sensation, language, and thought.

cerebrum   largest part of the brain of vertebrates, consisting of two hemispheres, whose function is to integrate sensory and neural activities and to facilitate learning and memory.

chromosome   structures found in the nucleus of most cells in an organism, on which genes are distributed and which divide and recombine as cells multiply. In humans, there are twenty-three matched pairs of chromosomes and one set of sex chromosomes in each somatic (body) cell; there are twenty-three pairs in germ cells (sperm and ova).

clone   an organism produced from a single ancestral cell, without sexual fertilization and containing the entire genetic complement of that ancestral cell.

differentiation of stem cells   the process whereby an unspecialized early embryonic cell acquires the features of a specialized cell such as a heart, liver, or muscle cell.

eugenics   the philosophy and study of improvement of characteristics in the human population by selective breeding among the more fit or the prevention of breeding of the less fit.

free will   the conscious activity of deliberate choice, involving reflection and evaluation of alternative courses of action.

gene   a unit of heredity, located on a chromosome, that produces a particular characteristic of the organism and made up of sequences of deoxyribonucleic acid (DNA).

genetic engineering   techniques to alter some function or element of an organism by inserting DNA from another organism.

genetic screening   the surveying of an entire population for a particular genetic mutation, a structural change in the sequence of DNA, associated with a particular disease, in the absence of particular signs and symptoms of disease, in order to find carriers.

institutional review board (IRB)   a group of scientists and laypersons formed by a research institution, under law, to review and approve research involving human subjects. In Britain, this body is called an ethics review committee (ERC).

neuron   a nerve cell, adapted to carry electrochemical impulses, by way of connections (synapses) throughout the body.

pluripotent stem cell   a single stem cell that has the capability of developing cells of all germ layers of an organism (endoderm, ectoderm, and mesoderm).

reproductive cloning   the creating of a clone by transfer of the nucleus of one organism into an ovum from which the nucleus has been removed and inserting it into the uterus of a female to carry to birth.

research   the planned and systematic search for new knowledge, utilizing methods to assure the validity of information, such as randomization (dividing the test subjects into two randomly selected but comparable groups), double-blinding (neither researcher nor recipient know what intervention is being given), and statistical analysis of results.

somatic cell nuclear transfer   the transfer of a cell nucleus from a somatic cell into an egg from which the nucleus has been removed.

stem cell   an undifferentiated cell that has the ability to divide for indefinite periods in culture and to give rise to specialized cells of the organism. Stem cells are found in the very early embryo, in which case they are capable of developing into all cells of the developed organism (*pluripotent*) or in certain tissues, such as bone marrow, in which case they develop into particular cell types, such as blood or muscle cells.

therapeutic cloning   research involving the creation of clones by nuclear transfer in order to attempt to proliferate and differentiate cell types for transplantation.

After Part IV

biodiversity   the variety of life at all levels of biological organization, including the diversity within a species (genetic), between species, and among ecosystems, due to evolution and environmental differences.

chemical, material, and energy cycles   The circular exchange of materials that is a basic component of the biosphere. Major cycles include the hydrological cycle, carbon cycle, and nitrogen cycle.

conservation   the preservation, protection, and management of the natural environment, together with the natural resources found therein, so that it will continue to exist in a fully functioning, intact, and healthy state into future generations. Conservation may also refer to the frugal use of water, heat, electricity, gas, and extracted minerals.

cultural relativism   the thesis that the moralty of cultures differ among themselves and that no normative value should be attached to any culture whereby comparative judgments of better and worse can be made.

cultural universals   certain practices that appear to exist, even in different forms, within all cultures, in order to sustain essential elements of human existence and communal cohesion (e.g., rules regarding sexual relationships and procreation and sanctions against killing).

culture   the complex of customs, values, and ways of life characteristic of a community sharing a historical tradition.

ecosystem   "Any entity or natural unit that includes living and nonliving parts interacting to produce a stable system in which the exchange of materials between living and nonliving parts follows circular paths is an ecological system or ecosystem" (Howard Odum). The ecosystem is a fundamental unit in ecology, allowing us to study and attempt to understand the interaction between geology, climate, and communities of organisms.

environment   the conditions under which any person or thing lives or is developed; the sum total of influences that modify and determine the development of life or character (*Oxford English Dictionary*).

genetically modified organisms (GMOs)   organisms into which segments of DNA from another species have been inserted to facilitate growth, resistance to infection, and tolerance of adverse conditions.

macro- and microallocation   the planning and processes whereby scarce resources are distributed over a large population (macro) or among a finite number of recipients (micro).

Index

208   *Index*

Oregon: assisted suicide, 56; rationing
    of health services, 151–52
organs. *See* donation of tissue

paternalism, 41, 44, 60
Percival, Thomas, 191
phrenology, 115
physician assisted suicide. *See*
    euthanasia
Plato, 12, 104, 181
Potter, van Rensselaer, 9, 140
preimplantation genetic diagnosis. *See*
    genetics
President's Commission for the Study of
    Ethical Problems in Medicine, 32,
    103, 107
President's Council on Bioethics, 134,
    150
Prometheus, 195, 197

quality of life, 35–36, 38, 39
Quinlan, Karen Ann, 33, 35–39

Raël, 127, 128
Ramsey, Paul, 3, 16; on abortion, 79; on
    eugenics, 106; on transplantation, 61
rationing of health care, 150–51
Rawls, John, 149
reductionism, 120
regenerative medicine, 130, 135
relativism, ethical, 155–57
research, 86–95; animals, 160, 163–65;
    children, women, 93; ethics of,
    89–91; public policy, 92; in genetics,
    93; international, 158
respect for persons, 17, 41–42, 89, 92;
    for fetus, embryo 71, 135
responsibility. *See* free will
reproduction, 67–76; artificial
    insemination, 69; assisted (ART),
    67; Human Fertilization and
    Embryology Authority, 71, 133; In
    vitro fertilization, 67–68, 71–72,
    130
Ricoeur, Paul, 116–17, 125

rights, 162–63; animal, 162
right to health care, 148–49
Rolston, Holmes, 173

sanctity of life, 38, 190
Santillán, Jésica, 59–60
Schiavo, Terri, 26–27, 33, 37, 39
Shelley, Mary, 9, 194–95, 197
Singer, Peter, 20, 162, 163
Socrates, 12, 124, 181, 186
stem cells, 130–38; defined, 130;
    embryonic and adult stem cells, 130
sterilization, 105
stoics, 12, 182, 183
suicide, 49–50, 51, 56
surrogate: decision maker, 44; mother,
    72–73

therapeutic equipoise. *See* clinical
    equipoise
totality, principle of, 61
transplantation, 59–66; donation, gift
    relationship, 63; presumed
    permission, 63; uniform anatomical
    gift act, 62; xenotransplantation, 64
triage, 8
Tuskegee syphilis study, 88

utilitarianism, 13, 162, 183–84; animal
    research, 162, 165; in environmental
    ethics, 169–71; in human research,
    89–90; utilitarianism vs.
    egalitarianism, 145

Veatch, Robert, 31, 36
vegetative state, 26, 27, 30, 35, 38;
    persistent, permanent, 30
vivisection, 164

Warnock, G. J., 13, 156, 178, 186
Warnock, Mary, 71
Watson, James, 98
Wexler, Nancy, 96, 97
Wilson, Edward O., 173, 175
Winslade, William, 122

About the Author

Albert Jonsen is one of the founders of the field of bioethics. He inaugurated instruction in medical ethics at University of California School of Medicine, San Francisco, in 1972 and headed the Department of Medical History and Ethics at the University of Washington School of Medicine. He served on two presidential commissions on bioethics. He is author of *The Birth of Bioethics* and *A Short History of Medical Ethics* and coauthor of *Clinical Ethics*. The American Society of Bioethics and Humanities bestowed on him its Lifetime Achievement Award.